ALLERGIES AND INFECTIOUS DISEASES

FOOD ALLERGY

ALEXANDER K. C. LEUNG
AND
JAMES S. C. LEUNG

Novinka
Nova Science Publishers, Inc.
New York

LIBRARY OF CONGRESS CATALOGING-IN-PUBLICATION DATA

Available upon Request
ISBN: 978-1-61728-952-1

Published by Nova Science Publishers, Inc. ✛ *New York*

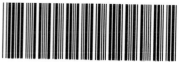
ALLERGIES AND INFECTIOUS DISEASES

FOOD ALLERGY

DATE DUE

ALLERGIES AND INFECTIOUS DISEASES

Additional books in this series can be found on Nova's website under the Series tab.

Additional E-books in this series can be found on Nova's website under the E-books tab.

FOOD AND BEVERAGE CONSUMPTION AND HEALTH

Additional books in this series can be found on Nova's website under the Series tab.

Additional E-books in this series can be found on Nova's website under the E-books tab.

CONTENTS

PREFACE

Food allergy is an adverse reaction resulting from an inappropriate immunological response to a food antigen. It usually presents as multi-system involvement. Gastrointestinal symptoms, cutaneous symptoms, and respiratory symptoms occur in 50 to 80%, 20 to 40%, and 4 to 25% of cases, respectively. Gastrointestinal manifestations include oral allergy syndrome, gastrointestinal anaphylaxis, allergic eosinophilic esophagitis, allergic eosinophilic gastro-enteropathy, food protein-induced enteropathy, food protein-induced entero-colitis syndrome, food protein-induced proctocolitis, gluten-sensitive enteropathy, infantile colic, irritable bowel syndrome, and constipation. Cutaneous manifestations are urticaria/angioedema, atopic dermatitis, contact dermatitis, and dermatitis herpetiformis. Finally, rhinitis/rhinoconjunctivitis, asthma, Heiner syndrome, and serous otitis media are the respiratory manifestations of food allergy. Other manifestations include systemic ana-phylaxis, food-dependent exercise-induced anaphylaxis, migraine, epilepsy, diabetes mellitus, nephrotic syndrome, nocturnal enuresis, anemia, thrombo-cytopenia, vasculitis, and arthropathy/arthritis.

Skin-prick testing with food extracts is often used to screen patients with suspected IgE-mediated food allergies. Simultaneously, since many children with IgE-mediated food allergies have elevated serum IgE levels, serum IgE antibodies specific for allergens can be measured in vitro by RAST, ELISA, or FEIA techniques. However, the double-blind placebo-controlled food challenge is objective and is considered the "gold standard" for the diagnosis of a food allergy. Nonetheless, an open or single-blind food challenge is acceptable when the resulting symptoms can be objectively observed. Definitive treatment of food allergy is strict elimination of the offending food from the diet. Symptomatic reactivity to food allergens is generally very specific, and patients rarely react to more than one food in a botanical or animal species. If elimination diets are prescribed, care must be taken to ensure that they are palatable and nutritionally adequate. Patients must have a good knowledge of foods containing the allergen and must be taught to scrutinize the labels of all packaged food carefully. Emergency treatment of food-induced anaphylaxis centers on basic life support principles, and intramuscular injection of epinephrine. A fast-acting H_1 antihistamine should be considered for the child with progressive or generalized urticaria or disturbing pruritus. Pharmacological therapies such as mast cell stabilizers have little role in the treatment of food allergy.

AUTHOR'S CONTACT INFORMATION

Alexander K. C. Leung
MBBS, FRCPC, FRCP(UK & Irel), FRCPCH, FAAP;
Clinical Professor of Pediatrics; The University of Calgary;
Pediatric Consultant;
Alberta Children's Hospital

James S. C. Leung
MD; Pediatric Resident; Hospital for Sick Children;
The University of Toronto

Chapter 1

INTRODUCTION

Food allergy (food hypersensitivity) is an adverse reaction resulting from an inappropriate immunological response to an antigen contained in food or food additive [1-5]. The reaction occurs in susceptible patients, and may be independent of the quantity of the offending substance ingested. Food allergy should be distinguished from food intolerance (nonallergic food hyper-sensitivity), which is an adverse reaction to food resulting from unique physiologic characteristic of the host, such as a metabolic disorder (e.g., lactase deficiency) [6]. Food toxicity is a separate entity resulting from effects of toxic contaminant or ingredient in food that effect healthy individuals in sufficient doses [6].

Chapter 2

EPIDEMIOLOGY

In the United States, up to 25% of adults self-report having a food allergy, and up to 25% of households report alteration of household dietary for individuals with perceived food allergies [7]. However, in developed contries, the prevalence of true, immunologically mediated food allergy is estimated to be 4 to 8% in children less than five years old [5-7]. The prevalence decreases after 5 years of age, such that an estimated 1 to 4% of adults in developed countries have food allergies [7]. These data reflect the general tendency for children to develop immunologic or "oral" tolerance to their food allergens with advancing age [5]. Approximately 85% of children with IgE mediated food allergies lose their food hypersensitivity by 3 to 5 years of age [8]. However, this natural history will vary with the specific food allergen. For example, cow's milk protein allergy that develops within the first year of life, resolves spontaneously in 80% of cases by age five years [9]. This is contrasted with peanut allergies that develop in childhood but resolve in approximately 20% of cases by adulthood [10]. New onset food allergies during adulthood are rare [7].

In young children, the most frequently implicated foods include eggs, cow's milk, tree nut, peanut, soy, wheat, seafood, citrus fruits, and chocolate [7]. In comparison, shellfish, peanuts, fish and tree nut allergies are frequently seen in adults as they are rarely outgrown [7]. Although often suspected, wheat and soy allergies are traditionally difficult to prove [7]. Geographic clustering of particular food allergies with particular populations has been noted [7].

In recent years, there is controversy regarding an increasing prevalence of specific food allergies in specific populations [7]. Although surveillance has increased in recent years, there is now clear evidence supporting and increased incidence of food allergy [11]. Evidence with peanuts is particularly compelling, with prospective studies from the United States and United Kingdom reporting a doubling in the prevalence of peanut allergies in young children over the last ten years [12,13]. Not surprisingly, this controversy has garnered significant media attention, and despite strong research initiatives, the precise etiology and rationale for these changes remains unclear [11].

Chapter 3

PATHOGENESIS

In the majority of cases, food allergies result from an IgE-mediated immune response. However, non-IgE-mediated responses may also occur. IgE-mediated reactions are caused by inflammatory mediators and cytokines released when food-derived antigens that are absorbed into blood, bind onto specific IgE residing on the surface of mast cells and basophils as well as lymphocytes, platelets, eosinophils and macrophages [14]. This binding results in release of histamine, heparin, prostaglandins, tryptase and leukotrienes which when act systemically inducing vasodilatation, mucus secretion, smooth muscle dilation [15]. These reactions are associated with rapid development of symptoms, usually within minutes to 2 hours, although late phase reactions from IgE-mediated cytokines may occur [14].

On the other hand, non-IgE reactions develop over hours, days or even weeks after exposure to food allergen [16]. The pathogenesis of these reactions is far less understood, with insufficient evidence to support type III (immune complex mediated) or type IV (cell-mediated) as exclusive processes [5]. This lack of understanding is partly due to the delayed onset of symptoms combined with lack of efficiency in making diagnosis once suspected [16]. Non-IgE reactions primarily affect the gut, and are histologically characterized by intense eosinophilic infiltration of the specific organ involved and may lead to chronic disorders such as allergic eosinophilic gastroenteropathy [16]. These reactions cause significant morbidity, but rarely mortality in patients [16].

In recent years, studies have focused on understanding the molecular pathogenesis, natural history and the recent increase in prevalence of food allergies. Specifically, a number of studies have queried the predisposition of young children towards food allergy, followed by their subsequent resolution with age. Understanding these fundamental mechanisms is believed by many to be a key to developing novel therapies and addressing the increasing incidence of food allergy [11]. At present, it is believed that a complex interplay of factors including:

- An immature gut mucosa in infants permitting increased absorption of intact food antigens.
- An immature immune system, especially at the gut mucosal level in infants unable to differentiate between innocent food allergens /nutrients, symbiotic gut flora and virulent microbes. Aging allows immunologic tolerance to develop and hence resolution of symptoms with age.
- Specific food allergens that elicit greater immunologic response.
- Genetic polymorphisms in particular populations that react immune-logically to particular food allergens.

Although the specific details and proposed molecular interactions with these hypotheses is beyond the scope of this clinically-oriented paper, excellent reviews on this topic were recently published by Cocharane et al and Jyonouchi [11,16].

Chapter 4

CLINICAL MANIFESTATIONS

Food allergies typically present with multi-system involvement. From a clinical and diagnostic perspective, it is helpful to subdivide clinical manifestations according to the predominant organ system(s) involved. Gastrointestinal symptoms occur most commonly with a frequency between 50 and 80% of cases, followed by cutaneous symptoms occurring in 20 to 40% and respiratory symptoms occurring in 4 to 25% of cases, respectively [14]. Symptoms may be mild or severe and most often occur within one to two hours after the offending food has been eaten. Occasionally, the onset of symptoms may be delayed for 48 to 72 hours.

Table 1. Clinical Manifestations of Food Allergy

Generalized manifestations	Systemic anaphylaxis
	Food-dependent exercise-induced anaphylaxis
Gastrointestinal manifestations	Oral allergy syndrome
	Gastrointestinal anaphylaxis
	Allergic eosinophilic esophagitis
	Allergic eosinophilic gastroenteropathy
	Food protein-induced enteropathy
	Food protein-induced enterocolitis syndrome
	Food protein-induced proctocolitis
	Gluten-sensitive enteropathy
	Infantile colic
	Irritable bowel syndrome
	Recurrent abdominal pain
	Constipation

Table 1. (Continued).

Cutaneous manifestations	Urticaria/angioedema
	Atopic dermatitis
	Contact dermatitis
	Dermatitis herpetiformis
Respiratory manifestations	Rhinitis/rhinoconjunctivitis
	Chronic sinusitis
	Asthma
	Heiner syndrome
	Serous otitis media
	Ménière's disease
Neurologic manifestations	Migraine
	Epilepsy
Endocrine manifestation	Diabetes mellitus
Renal manifestations	Nephrotic syndrome
Hematologic manifestations	Anemia
	Thrombocytopenia
Rheumatic manifestation	Vasculitis
	Arthropathy/arthritis

GENERALIZED MANIFESTATIONS

Systemic Anaphylaxis

Systemic anaphylaxis secondary to ingestion of food allergen is potentially fatal, and the most common cause of anaphylaxis treated in emergency departments [6]. However, overall, systemic anaphylaxis is an uncommon manifestation of food allergy [17]. Systemic anaphylaxis usually occurs within minutes, but occasionally hours after the ingestion of an offending food [18]. Peanuts, nuts, eggs, and seafood are responsible for the majority of these reactions [19]. Early symptoms may include pruritis, "metallic" taste in the mouth, sensation of tightness in the throat, flushing, urticaria, dizziness, nausea, vomiting, abdominal pain, angioedema, and wheezing [20]. This may rapidly progress to laryngeal edema, dyspnea, stridor, diaphoresis, cyanosis, chest pain, hypotension, cardiac dysrhythmias, and shock [21,22]. The degree of anaphylactic reactions varies and may be manifested in a partial form. In general, the more rapidly anaphylaxis occurs after exposure to an offending agent, the more likely the anaphylactic reaction is to be severe and potentially life-threatening [19]. Anaphylactic reactions to foods can be biphasic with an early and late phase separated by one to eight hours or there may be multiple recurrences separated by asymptomatic periods lasting for hours [14,23]. Some very severe anaphylactic reactions are protracted and last continuously for many hours without remission [14]. Risk factors for severe anaphylactic reactions include history of a previous anaphylactic reaction, history of poorly controlled asthma, allergy to peanuts, nuts and shellfish, and use of ß-blockers or acetycholinesterase inhibitors [4,24]. Low levels of serum platelet-activating factor acetylhydrolase may be a marker for more severe food-induced anaphylaxis [24].

Food-Dependent Exercise-Induced Anaphylaxis

Anaphylaxis has been reported after the ingestion of foods in association with exercise [25-27]. Food-dependent exercise-induced anaphylaxis represents 7 to 9% of anaphylactic reactions [28]. The condition is twice as common in females and 60% of cases occur in individuals under the age of 30 years [24,28]. There is often a history of atopy [28]. One subset of patients may develop anaphylaxis in temporal proximity to ingestion of any type of food [20,29]. The other subset may develop anaphylaxis with exercise in conjunction with ingestion of a specific food [20]. The latter subset is more common than the former subset [20]. Foods associated with food-specific exercise-induced anaphylaxis include crustaceans, celery, grapes, tomato, wheat, buckwheat, chicken, and dairy products [29,30]. Rarely, two foods have to be eaten together to provoke an anaphylactic attack [31]. When each food is taken separately, food-dependent exercise-induced anaphylaxis does not occur [31]. Typical symptoms include urticaria, angioedema, dyspnea, and abdominal pain [32]. These may progress to hypotension and shock. Loss of consciousness is seen in approximately 30% of cases [32].

Although various exercises may lead to anaphylaxis in susceptible individuals, jogging is the exercise most frequently reported, followed by aerobics and walking [28,29,33]. Anaphylaxis usually occurs when exercise takes place within two to four hours of food ingestion [20]. Unlike exercise-induced anaphylaxis, anaphylactic symptoms develop only in the presence of both food ingestion and exercise [34]. Food-dependent exercise-induced anaphylaxis often presents with scalp pruritis prior to systemic symptoms [20].

The exact mechanism of food-dependent exercise-induced anaphylaxis is not known. There is evidence of IgE-mediated sensitization to the food allergen [28]. Skin testing may show an immediate flare-and-wheal reaction to the implicated food [27]. Blood flow differences to the gut, increased food allergen absorption, increased spontaneous leukocyte histamine release, lowered mast cell releasability threshold, and enhanced mast cell responsiveness to physical stimuli may have a role in the pathogenesis of this condition [27,29,33].

GASTROINTESTINAL MANIFESTATIONS

Oral Allergy Syndrome

Oral allergy syndrome (pollen-food allergy syndrome) is a complex of symptoms induced by exposure of the oral and pharyngeal mucosa to plant protein allergens [35,36]. Patients are usually sensitized to an aeroallergen initially [35]. The IgE antibodies to the aeroallergen cause the oral allergy syndrome [37]. Botanical cross-reactivity as a result of shared epitopes between pollen and causative fruits and vegetables has been suggested as a possible mechanism of local mast cell activation [38]. The oral allergy syndrome is considered a form of contact urticaria that is confined mainly to the oropharynx [5]. Symptoms include rapid onset of itching, tingling, burning, and/or angioedema of the lips, tongue, palate, and throat within minutes of ingestion of fresh fruit and vegetable [36]. Symptoms usually resolve rapidly. Occasionally, the clinical course is more dramatic with potentially fatal pharyngeal swelling or progression towards a generalized anaphylactic reaction [14,39]. The syndrome generally occurs in patients with inhalant allergy to birch, mugwort, or ragweed pollen and is associated with the ingestion of various fresh fruits (e.g., apples, bananas, melons, citrus fruits) and raw vegetables (e.g. carrots, tomatoes, celery) [40-43]. It is uncommon to have several fruits and vegetables that cause the oral allergy syndrome in one patient [44]. However, cross-reactivity with different fruits processing homologous protein segments has been described [45]. Oral allergy syndrome is more prevalent in adults than in children [46]. Most patients have some degree of allergic conjunctivitis or allergic rhinitis because the IgE antibodies to an aeroallergen cross-react with the fruit or vegetable proteins [35,47]. It is interesting to note that if the offending fruit or vegetable is cooked, then the patient does not usually experience any symptom as the food allergens are generally denatured by heating [35]. Patients who remain sensitive to cooked fruit or vegetable may be sensitive to proteins that do not cross-react with pollens and do not actually have oral allergy syndrome [42,48]. Although these patients react to food typically associated with oral allergy syndrome, the absence of pollenosis and presence of symptoms beyond the oropharynx suggest conventional food allergy rather than oral allergy syndrome [42].

Gastrointestinal Anaphylaxis

Gastrointestinal anaphylaxis is an IgE-mediated gastrointestinal hypersensitivity that often accompanies other systemic manifestations of food allergy [49]. This may be manifested as nausea, vomiting, abdominal pain, flatulence, abdominal distension, or diarrhea [5]. The reaction usually occurs within minutes to 2 hours of food ingestion [50]. Repeated ingestion of a food allergen may induce partial desensitization of mast cells in the gastrointestinal tract resulting in milder symptoms [5,39].

Allergic Eosinophilic Esophagitis

Allergic eosinophilic esophagitis is characterized by intense eosinophilic infiltration of the esophageal mucosa (>20 eosinophils per high-power field) and severe basal cell hyperplasia [51-54]. However, First International Gastrointestinal Eosinophil Research Symposium Subcommittees (FIGERS) recently suggested that the presence of 15 eosinophils in esophageal mucosa is sufficient to establish the diagnosis of eosinophilic esophagitis [55].

The condition is usually T-cell-mediated rather than IgE-mediated, and caused by allergens in the diet and, less commonly, in the air [52,54,56-58]. Allergic eosinophilic esophagitis occurs mainly in children and young adults [59-60]. This condition is being more frequently diagnosed over the past decade. The condition is more common in males and those with a family or personal history of atopy or proven food allergy [53,61]. Allergic eosinophilic esophagitis may present with irritability, sleep disturbance, food refusal, vomiting/ regurgitation, dysphagia, abdominal pain, substernal chest pain, occult blood loss, anemia, and failure to thrive [41,51,54,55]. Dauer et al retrospectively reviewed the records of 71 children with biopsy-proven allergic eosinophilic esophagitis and found that the most common symptom was dysphagia, being present in 36 (51%) patients [51]. Eighteen (50%) of the 36 patients with dysphagia experienced at least one episode of food impaction. Other common symptoms include vomiting (31%) and abdominal pain (24%). The symptoms of recurrent vomiting /regurgitation may mimic those of gastroesophageal reflux but are refractory to anti-reflux treatment [55,62,63]. These symptoms respond to dietary avoidance of food allergens [63].

Allergic Eosinophilic Gastroenteropathy

Allergic eosinophilic gastroenteritis is characterized by infiltration of the gastrointestinal tract with eosinophils, peripheral eosinophilia, and absence of vasculitis [64,65]. The eosinophilic infiltrates may be quite patchy and may involve the mucosa, muscular layer, or serosal layer of the stomach or small intestine [29,45].

Although allergic eosinophilic gastroenteropathy may affect individuals of all ages, the disease is more common in individuals in the third through fifth decades of life [64]. Patients with mucosal involvement usually have postprandial nausea, vomiting, abdominal pain, watery diarrhea with or without blood, iron deficiency anemia, occasionally steatorrhea, and weight loss in adults or failure to thrive in children [21,29,66]. Patients with muscular involvement may have symptoms and signs of gastric outlet or intestinal obstruction, depending on the site of bowel involvement [45]. The serosal form is characterized by ascites, abdominal pain, and abdominal distension and is extremely rare in children [45,67].

Food Protein-Induced Enteropathy

Food protein-induced enteropathy is characterized by protracted diarrhea and vomiting with onset usually in infancy. This may result in malabsorption, protein-losing enteropathy, and failure to thrive [42,50]. The disorder is caused by a T-cell-mediated response most commonly to cow's milk protein [45]. Intestinal biopsy typically reveals a patchy villous atrophy, increased crypt length, and prominent mononuclear round cell infiltrates [68].

Food Protein-Induced Enterocolitis Syndrome

Food protein-induced enterocolitis syndrome is a cell-mediated hypersensitivity disease that occurs mainly in infants under 3 months of age [69]. The condition usually resolves by 2 years of age but may, rarely, persist into late childhood [46]. Cow's milk and soy protein are most often responsible [41,53,67], other food antigens have occasionally been implicated [7]. Classic symptoms are protracted vomiting and diarrhea [29,50,70]. Additional signs and symptoms include irritability, lethargy, anemia, transient methemo-globinemia, abdominal distension, protein-losing enteropathy, and failure to thrive [42,45,70-72]. Stools generally contain occult blood, poly-morphonuclear neutrophils, eosinophils, and Charcot-Leyden crystals [5]. Presumably, stimulation of T-cells by food allergens with secretion of tumor necrosis factor-α may play a role in the pathophysiology of this disorder [50,70,73]. A relative lack of expression of transforming growth factor-β may also have a role to play [70,73]. Skin tests for the offending antigen are usually negative [46]. Radioallergosorbent (RAST) assay, which detects specific IgE antibody, may also be negative in these patients. Jejunal biopsy specimens usually reveal villus atrophy and increased numbers of lymphocytes, eosinophils, and mast cells [29,74]. Colonoscopy and biopsy show inflammatory colitis and eosinophilic infiltration [75]. Symptoms usually resolve in 72 hours after the offending food substance has been removed from the diet.

Food Protein-Induced Proctocolitis

As with food protein-induced enterocolitis syndrome, food protein-induced proctocolitis is a T-cell mediated disorder. The disorder usually occurs in the first few months of life and is most often secondary to milk protein or soy protein hypersensitivity [67,74]. Unlike food protein-induced enterocolitis syndrome, infants with food protein-induced proctocolitis generally appear healthy and have normal weight gain. These infants usually have occult or gross blood and occasionally mucus in their stools but classically, do not have diarrhea [50,76,77]. In breastfed infants, elimination of food-allergen from the maternal diet may result in resolution of hematochezia. In general, hematochezia resolves within 72 hours of appropriate food-allergen avoidance [50]. Colonic biopsy samples reveal mucosal edema, erythema, friability, ulceration, nodular lymphoid hyperplasia and eosinophilic infiltration [29,78]. However, colonic biopsy findings are often nonspecific and unhelpful as the disease of focal in nature and require sampling from the appropriate sites [79]. The diagnosis is primarily clinical as laboratory tests are generally unreliable [79]. Food challenges are also helpful [79].

Gluten-Sensitive Enteropathy

Gluten-sensitive enteropathy, or celiac disease, is a disorder in which small-bowel mucosal damage is the result of a permanent sensitivity to gliadin, the alcohol-soluble portion of gluten, present in wheat, barley, and rye. Patients with gluten-sensitive enteropathy classically present with diarrhea/ steatorrhea, abdominal distension, muscle wasting, and failure to thrive [4]. Other clinical manifestations include irritability, anorexia, vomiting, abdominal pain, oral ulcers, digital clubbing, delayed puberty, and infertility [80,81]. However, patients with gluten-sensitive enteropathy may be asymptomatic [81]. The presence of anti-gliadin, anti-endomysial, and anti-tissue transglutaminase of the IgA isotype and anti-gliadin of the IgG isotype support the diagnosis [42]. However, anti-gliadin antibody of IgG subtype has been known to be positive in conditions such as cow's milk protein allergy, inflammatory bowel disease, and cystic fibrosis and therefore has poor specificity. In addition, patients with IgA deficiency may not have antibodies of IgA subtype in spite of suffering from gluten-sensitive enteropathy. It is recommended that the diagnosis of gluten-sensitive enteropathy be confirmed by intestinal biopsy before instituting dietary changes. Characteristically, biopsy of the jejunum shows villus atrophy, marked increase in crypt-villous ratio, and extensive cellular infiltrates [29]. Both cellular and complement-mediated cytotoxicity and lymphokine-induced damage have been implicated in the pathogenesis of the condition [63]. There is a genetic predisposition to the disease. There is a predominance of certain HLA types (B8, DQ2, DW3) in patients with gluten-sensitive enteropathy [4,5]. Environmental factors may influence expression of the genetic predisposition

Infantile Colic

There is increasing evidence that cow's milk proteins may play a role in infantile colic [82-88]. Approximately 25% of infants with moderate or severe colic have allergy to cow's milk protein [89,90]. Lothe and Lindberg showed that colic disappeared in 24 of 27 infants when they were given a cow's milk-free diet [86]. These infants were entered into a double-blind placebo-controlled crossover trial of whey protein. Eighteen infants receiving the whey protein capsules reacted with colic, two infants received placebo reacted with colic, and four infants did not react at all.

Iacono et al put 70 cow's milk formula-fed infants with severe colic on soy-milk formula [84]. In 50 infants, there was a remission of symptoms when cow's milk protein was eliminated from their diet. Two successive challenges caused the return of symptoms in all these 50 infants. Follow-ups, after an average period of 18 months, showed that in 22 of 50 (44%) of the infants who had cow's milk protein-related colic and 1 of 20 (5%) of those with non-cow's milk protein-related colic developed an overt form of alimentary intolerance. Lucassen et al randomly selected 43 healthy infants with colic to receive whey hydrolysate formula or standard formula [87]. They found a decrease in the duration of crying in those infants fed with whey hydrolysate formula.

Jakobsson et al studied the effectiveness of 2 formulae with extensively hydrolysed casein in 22 infants with severe colic [91]. One infant was considered as treatment failure and six infants as protocol failures. The remaining 15 infants showed a significant decrease in the lengths of time they cried as well as a decrease in the intensity of their crying on both formulae. When the infants were challenged in a double-blind design, 11 infants reacted with an increase in crying time to cow's milk protein or bovine whey protein.

Hill et al studied the effect of diet change in 38 bottle-fed and 77 breast-fed colicky infants in a double-blind, randomized, placebo-controlled trial [83]. Bottle-fed infants were assigned to either casein hydrolysate or cow's milk formula. All mothers of breast-fed infants were started on an artificial color-free, preservative-free, additive-free diet and were randomized to receive either an active low allergen (milk free) diet or a control diet. Hill et al showed that infants on the active diet had their distress reduced by 39% compared with 16% for those on the control diet.

Jakobsson and Lindberg put 66 mothers of 66 breast-fed infants with infantile colic on a cow's milk-free diet [92]. The colic disappeared in 35 infants; it reappeared after reintroduction of cow's milk into the mother's diet in 23 of the 35 infants. A double-blind crossover trial with cow's milk whey protein was performed in 16 of these 23 mothers and infants. Six infants had to be taken out of the study for various reasons. Of the remaining 10 infants, nine displayed signs of colic after their mothers had taken the whey-filled capsules.

Maternal ingestion of eggs, chocolate, citrus fruits, nuts, as well as certain seafood whilst breastfeeding may result in infantile colic [85,93,94]. Hill et al randomized mothers of 107 term breastfed infants younger than 6 weeks of age with colic to follow a low-allergen diet with elimination of dairy products, soy, wheat, eggs, peanuts, tree nuts, and fish (n=53) and a control group (n=54) whose diet contained the known allergen [95]. Forty seven mothers in the treatment group and 43 mothers in the control group completed the study.

Infants were identified as responders if there was at least 25% reduction in duration of crying/fussing on days 8 and 9. The authors showed that 74% of infants in the treatment group versus 37% of infants in the control group were responders (p=<0.001).

Irritable Bowel Syndrome

The pathogenesis of irritable colon syndrome is likely heterogeneous. Food allergy has been implicated in the pathogenesis of a subset of patients with irritable bowel syndrome [96,97]. The association of irritable bowel syndrome with specific IL-10 genotypes supports involvement of the immune system in its pathogenesis [71,98,99]. Patients with irritable bowel syndrome have a greater area of intestinal mucosa occupied by mast cells than do healthy control individuals [100]. A study of dietary eliminations in patients with irritable bowel syndrome found a significant reduction in symptom score in those patients whose exclusions were guided by raised IgG antibodies to dietary antigens than did patients on a sham diet based on irrelevant antigens [101]. Reintroduction of eliminated foods resulted in aggravation of symptoms in patients whose dietary exclusions were guided by raised IgG antibodies to dietary antigens. Irritable bowel syndrome might result from an interplay between immunological dysfunction, impaired gut barrier functions, susceptible genes and other environmental factors [102]. It has been hypothesized that food antigens induce mast cells to secrete mediators that regulate gastrointestinal motility and pain perception through gastrointestinal neural system [96].

Recurrent Abdominal Pain

Recurrent abdominal pain is usually defined as three or more bouts of abdominal pain, severe enough to interfere with a child's normal activities, occurring over a period of not less than three months during the year preceding the examination [103,104]. Onset often occurs between five and 10 years of age. Typically, the pain is vague, poorly localized or periumbilical and may be crampy or sharp. Episodes of pain tend to cluster, alternating with pain-free periods of variable length [104]. Most episodes last for less than an hour. On cessation of the pain, the child is up and about as if nothing had happened. In the majority of cases, the cause is functional [104,105]. Organic causes account for 5 to 10% of cases [103,104]. Kokkonen et al studied 84 children with recurrent abdominal pain [105]. Food allergy was diagnosed in 28 (33%) children based on an open elimination challenge test. However, the study was criticized because a formal diagnosis would require a double-blind placebo-controlled food challenge [106]. Further studies using double-blind placebo-controlled food challenges are necessary before food allergy can be established as a cause of recurrent abdominal pain in children.

Constipation

The vast majority of constipation in children is functional [107,108]. Constipation resulting from IgE sensitization to cow's milk has been described [108]. Loening-Baucke reviewed the records of 4157 children between 0 to 24 months of age seen in general pediatric clinics for health maintenance and acute care visits [108]. Of the 185 children with constipation, food allergy was responsible for constipation in only 2 (1%) of these children [108]. In contrast, Iacono et al studied 27 consecutive infants with chronic "idiopathic" constipation and noted improvement or resolution of symptoms in 21(78%) of these infants after a 4-week period of a cow's milk-free diet [109]. These infants had a relapse of symptoms on cow's milk challenge. Iacono et al subsequently performed a randomized cross-over trial of a cow's milk-based diet versus a soy milk-based diet in 65 children with chronic constipation [110]. Forty-four (68%) of the 65 children had increased bowel movements and improvement of fecal score while receiving the soy milk. None of the children who received cow's milk had a response. In all 44 children with a response, the response was confirmed with a double-blind challenge with cow's milk. Daher et al studied 25 children with chronic constipation [111]. In seven (28%) patients, the constipation disappeared while they were following a diet free of cow's milk protein and reappeared within 48 to 72 hours after challenge with cow's milk. In two patients, a rectal biopsy revealed allergic colitis with eosinophilic infiltration and they therefore did not undergo the challenge. High serum levels of total IgE were observed in five (71%) of the seven patients who showed a clinical improvement. Two (29%) patients had a positive skin test and two (29%) had detectable levels of specific IgE. Carroccio et al treated 52 children with chronic constipation unresponsive to common treatment by exclusion of milk alone, or by an extensive oligoallergenic diet if unresponsive [112]. Twenty four patients were found to be suffering from cow's milk intolerance and six from multiple food intolerance. These patients had a normal stool frequency on elimination diet with recurrence of constipation on food challenge. These patients showed a significantly higher frequency of mucosal erosions, number of intraepithelial lymphocytes and eosinophils, and number of eosinophils in the lamina propria. The remaining 22 patients did not respond to the elimination diet. Murch identified 30 children with constipation who responded to the exclusion diet with resolution of symptom; six of these children were allergic to multiple antigens [71]. Rectal biopsy of the affected patients showed eosinophilic proctitis [71]. Carroccio et al performed a Medline search for articles published between 1970 and June 2006, using the key words "chronic constipation or constipation" and "food intolerance or allergy". The authors identified 33 papers but only 19 of them were related to the topic. Analysis of these papers showed a relationship between constipation and food allergy in a subgroup of pediatric patients with "idiopathic" constipation unresponsive to laxative treatment. Additional studies are necessary to substantiate the specific associations and to clarify the pathogenic mechanisms involved.

CUTANEOUS MANIFESTATIONS

Urticaria/Angioedema

Acute urticaria and, to a lesser extent, angioedema are among the most common manifestations of food allergic reactions in children [21,29]. They tend to occur more commonly in younger patients and in atopic patients, in association with other systemic features [113]. Symptoms result from activation of IgE-bearing cells by circulating food allergens absorbed through the gastrointestinal tract. The foods most commonly incriminated include eggs, milk, peanuts, and nuts [114]. In several studies, urticaria/angioedema occurred in 10 to 15% of infants with challenge-proven milk allergy [115,116]. In a classic study of 554 adults with urticaria, food allergy was demonstrated as the cause in only 1.4% of cases [117].

Physical contact with foods may also cause acute urticaria [116,118,119]. Allergic contact urticaria can be seen in children who are sensitized to environmental allergens such as food or classically, latex allergy [120]. There is a potential for cross-reactivity with various foods in individuals with latex allergy [120]. Food allergy is rarely the cause of chronic urticaria, unless the offending food is eaten almost every day [21,29,49,113].

Atopic Dermatitis

Atopic dermatitis is a multifactorial disease, and food allergy is associated with 30 to 50% of young children who had moderate to severe atopic dermatitis [121-123]. Burks et al evaluated 46 patients who had atopic dermatitis from food hypersensitivity substantiated with double-blind placebo-controlled food challenges [124]. Sixty five food challenges were performed; 27 (42%) were interpreted as positive in 15 (33%) patients. Sampson et al studied 350 patients with severe atopic dermatitis for possible food hypersensitivity [49,125,126]. Food allergy was diagnosed by double-blind placebo-controlled food challenges. Cutaneous reactions developed in 75% of the positive challenges within minutes to two hours, but only 30% of the positive responses were isolated cutaneous symptoms alone [49]. Most of the skin manifestations consisted of a markedly pruritic, erythematous rash that developed in sites with a predilection for atopic dermatitis.

In a prospective study of 113 patients with atopic dermatitis, marked improvement was noted in those who were maintained on an allergen elimination diet when compared with a similar group of patients who did not have food allergy or who did not adhere to the elimination diet [125]. Breuer et al performed 106 double-blind placebo-controlled food challenges to cow's milk, egg, wheat, and soy on 64 children who had atopic dermatitis [127]. Twenty-eight (57%) of the 49 positive reactions resulted in late eczematous reactions, either as isolated events or in combination with immediate reactions. Hill et al evaluated 487 infants who had skin prick tests to cow's milk, egg, and peanut, and who had a family history of atopic dermatitis, asthma, or immediate food allergy in a parent or sibling [128]. One hundred and forty-one (28.9%) of these infants had atopic dermatitis by the age of 12 months. These authors found that as the severity of atopic dermatitis increased, so did the prevalence of IgE-mediated food allergy and also the frequency of adverse food allergy reactions. The relative risk of an infant who had atopic dermatitis to develop an IgE-mediated food allergy was 5.9 for the most severely affected group.

The pathogenesis of atopic dermatitis likely involves both immediate and late-phase effects of IgE-mediated food hypersensitivity reactions as well as cell-mediated reactions [21,49,118]. The immediate or early phase of the reaction results from IgE-mediated cutaneous mast cell activation [126]. The late phase is characterized by a mixed cellular infiltrate (eosinophils, neutrophils, lymphocytes, and basophils) at six to eight hours and thereafter by a mononuclear round cell infiltrate indistinguishable from that seen in eczematous skin [125,129,130]. The pattern of cytokine expression is predominantly that of the Th2 type, namely, interleukin-4, -5 and -13 [113,114]. A single ingestion of food allergen may not provoke an eczematous lesion, but chronic ingestion of a food allergen can result in the classic changes of atopic dermatitis [121]. Children who have atopic dermatitis and documented food allergy may develop typical eczematous lesions while the disease is active, but may develop urticaria with ingestion of a food allergen when the atopic dermatitis is in remission [123]. On the other hand, atopic dermatitis is also seen in patients with X-linked agammaglobulinemia, suggesting that, at least in some cases, atopic dermatitis is not IgE-mediated [131]. Testing for cow's milk allergy, Hill et al identified a delayed eczematous reaction in 17 of 135 children with atopic dermatitis [132]. Ten of the 17 children had negative prick test to cow's milk allergen, suggesting a non-IgE mediated pathogenesis. Lio suggests that there are at least two types of "food allergy" in patients with atopic dermatitis: the IgE-mediated immediate reactions and the cell-mediated eczematous reactions [131].

Contact Dermatitis

Contact dermatitis may be related to an immune-mediated reaction to food or a direct toxic effect of the food coming into contact with the skin [114,133]. Food-induced contact dermatitis is often seen among food handlers, especially those who handle raw shellfish and eggs [6,102,134]. Allergic contact cheilitis has been reported from the chewing of garlic [135] and from the contact of geraniol, a food additive contained in certain foods [136].

Dermatitis Herpetiformis

Gluten-sensitive enteropathy is found in 75 to 95% of patients with dermatitis herpetiformis [118,137]. Dermatitis herpetiformis is a cutaneous cell-mediated response to gliadin that is present in wheat, rye, and barley [29,114]. The disorder is characterized by a chronic, intensely pruritic, papulovesicular rash, symmetrically distributed over the extensor surfaces of the extremities and buttocks [68,114]. Approximately 80 to 90% of patients have the HLA-B8 haplotype, and more than 90% have the HLA-Dw3 haplotype [138]. Skin biopsy generally reveals granular and linear deposits of IgA, C3, as well as infiltrates with polymorphonuclear leukocytes.

Immunoglobulin A deposits may activate complement through the alternative pathway and cause inflammation. An IgE-mediated hypersensitivity reaction does not contribute to the pathogenesis. IgA antibodies to smooth muscle endomysium and jejunum have been reported in patients with dermatitis herpetiformis-associated gluten-sensitive enteropathy [118]. Also, antibodies to tissue transglutaminase and epidermal transglutaminase are present in patients with dermatitis herpetiformis, suggesting that epidermal transglutaminase is the autoantigen in dermatitis herpetiformis [114].

RESPIRATORY MANIFESTATIONS

Rhinitis/Rhinoconjunctivitis

Food-induced allergic rhinitis/rhinoconjunctivitis is more frequently observed in children than in adults [122,139]. Rhinitis/rhinoconjunctivitis following inhalation of food dusts or vapor is not uncommon in patients with food allergy [14]. Rhinitis/rhinoconjunctivitis typically occurs in association with other clinical manifestations such as cutaneous and/or gastrointestinal symptoms during acute allergic reactions to foods [40,140]. Rhinitis/rhinoconjunctivitis as the sole manifestation of food allergy is quite uncommon [49,67,135,139]. Allergic rhinitis may be manifested as nasal congestion, sneezing, and rhinorrhea [141]. Allergic conjunctivitis is characterized by periocular erythema, ocular injection, pruritis, and tearing. It seems likely that ingested allergens can activate nasal mast cells in addition to mast cells elsewhere in the body [141].

Chronic Sinusitis

Allergy to food allergens has been suggested to be a rare cause of chronic sinusitis [142]. Food allergy should be suspected in refractory cases of chronic sinusitis in which no apparent cause can be found, especially in atopic individuals with perennial symptoms [120,142].

Asthma (Bronchospasm)

Asthma from food allergy is a mixed IgE- and cell-mediated response due to the involvement of IgE antibodies, mast cells, eosinophils, and T-lymphocytes [42]. The condition occurs more often in children than in adults [143,144]. In several studies, 2 to 6% of children with asthma were found to have wheezing provoked by blinded food challenges [139,143-146]. Asthmatic children have a 14-fold higher risk of developing a severe allergic reaction to food compared with children without asthma [144,147].

In some children, food allergy may increase airway reactivity so that other triggers or environmental factors can more readily precipitate an asthmatic attack [148,149]. Vapors containing proteins emitted from cooking food can induce asthmatic attacks [6,143,150,151]. Inhalational exposures to foods, particular in the workplace, account for approximately 1% of asthmatic attacks in the adult population [6,149]. "Baker's asthma" caused by inhalation of flour or mold-derived enzymes used as flour additives are one such example [29]. Affected individuals have asthmatic attacks in association with exposure to aerosolized wheat proteins and have positive skin prick tests or serum specific IgE to wheat proteins [146,149]. Likewise, peanut dust in airplanes can provoke allergic reactions in susceptible individuals [152]. Allergenic proteins may also reach the respiratory tract via the circulation or they may act via inflammatory mediators released from the skin or gastrointestinal tract [149].

Food allergy in early infancy increases the risk for developing asthma in later life [144,153,154]. This applies also to children who have outgrown their food allergies [155].

Heiner Syndrome

Primary pulmonary hemosiderosis with hypersensitivity to cow's milk (Heiner syndrome) is a rare condition that usually occurs in young children. The syndrome is characterized by chronic cough, wheezing, hemoptysis, pulmonary infiltrates, hemosiderosis, gastrointestinal blood loss, iron deficiency anemia, and failure to thrive [139,156]. Presumably, the syndrome results from aspiration of milk into the lungs with subsequent development of IgG cow's milk antibodies and an immune complex Arthus-type reaction in the alveoli [157]. If the vasculitis is severe, alveolar bleeding and pulmonary hemosiderosis may result [157]. Affected children have usually high titers of precipitins to multiple constituents of cow's milk and positive results on intradermal skin tests to various cow's milk proteins [156]. Dietary elimination of cow's milk results in symptomatic improvement, and reintroduction of cow's milk results in recurrence of symptoms. It has been postulated that antigen-antibody complexes and cell-mediated hypersensitivity play a pathogenic role in this syndrome based on the presence of elevated serum levels of milk-specific IgG antibodies and the in vitro proliferative response of the patient's lymphocytes to milk antigen [141].

Serous Otitis Media

Serous otitis media, defined as non-purulent collection of fluid in the middle ear, is a multifactorial disease [158]. Food allergy may play a role in the pathogenesis in a subgroup of children with serous otitis media [159-161]. It has been hypothesized that allergic inflammation in the nasal mucosa may cause Eustachian tube dysfunction that may result in serous otitis media [140,160]. IgG complexes with cow's milk protein might also contribute to the middle ear inflammation [162]. In the study by Aydoğan et al, food allergy was detected in 25 (44.6%) of 56 patients with serous otitis media [158]. In patients with food allergy, serous otitis media was detected in 7 (25%) of 28 patients. In the control group of 28 patients, food allergy was diagnosed in 5 (18%) patients and serous otitis media in one (3%) patient. The incidence of food allergy in serous otitis media group was statistically significant when compared to the normal group. The risk of otitis media in children having food allergy was 3.7 times higher than the control. Bernstein et al evaluated 100 patients aged 2 to18 years with recurrent serous otitis media for IgE-mediated hypersensitivity [159]. Thirty five of these patients had allergic rhinitis. Total IgE was increased in the middle ear fluid in 16 of the 35 patients with allergic rhinitis and in only 2 of the 65 patients in the non-allergic group. In 8 of these 16 patients (23% of the allergic group), levels of IgE per milligram of protein were higher in the middle ear effusion than in the corresponding serum, thus suggesting local production of IgE by the middle ear mucosa in these patients. In a subset of infants with recurrent serous otitis media, IgG complexes with food antigen may contribute to middle ear inflammation and serous otitis media [150,162]. Nsouli et al evaluated 104 unselected children with recurrent serous otitis media for food allergy [161]. There was a significant statistical association, by chi-square analysis, between food allergy and recurrent serous otitis media in 81 (78%) of the 104 patients. An elimination diet led to a significant amelioration of serous otitis media in 70 (86%) of 81 patients. An open challenge diet with the suspected offending food(s) provoked a recurrence of serous otitis media in 66 (94%) of 70 patients. Further studies with double-blind placebo-controlled food challenge are necessary to confirm these findings.

Ménière's Disease

Ménière's disease is characterized by recurrent vertigo, fluctuating hearing loss, aural fullness or pressure, and tinnitus [163,164]. Derebery et al did a mail-survey on 1490 patients with Ménière's disease [163]. Of 734 respondents with Ménière's disease, 296 (40.3%) had or suspected food allergies and 272 (37%) had confirmatory skin or in vitro tests for allergy. These prevalence rates were significantly higher than those found in the control group of patients (n=172) with otologic problems other than Ménière's disease, of which 43 (25%) had or suspected food allergies and 38 (22.2%) had confirmatory skin or in vitro tests for allergy. Keleş et al studied 46 patients aged between 26 and 68 years and 46 aged-matched controls. The authors found that total serum IgE levels were above the normal levels in 19 (41.3%) of the patients with Ménière's disease and 9 (19.5%) of the controls [164]. A history of allergy was found in 31 (67.3%) of the patients with Ménière's disease and 16 (34.7%) of the controls. When the specific IgE levels were measured (all seasons, tree, fungus, fruit, egg white, cow's milk, wheat flour, corn flour, beef, and rice), the number of patients having all the panels negative was eight (17.9%) in patients with Ménière's disease and 31 (67.3%) in the controls. Cow's milk allergy was the most common identifiable cause of Ménière's disease. It has been hypothesized that immune complexes circulating in the blood might hinder the filtering ability of the endolymphatic sac [164].

NEUROLOGIC MANIFESTATIONS

Migraine

Medical consensus is that food allergy does not play a significant role in migraine [122]. Several double-blind studies have shown that some patients with migraine had adverse reactions to certain foods, as shown by dietary exclusion and subsequent challenge [165-167]. However, there was no clearly proven immunologic effect of food components in many of these patients [168]. Foods rich in tyramine, tryptamine, serotonin, and histamine can trigger migraine, and this is based mainly on pharmacologic rather than immunologic effects [169,170]. According to the revised nomenclature for allergy published by the European Academy of Allergy and Clinical Immunology, these kinds of adverse reactions are classified as toxic reactions rather than food hypersensitivity [171].

Epilepsy

Associations between epilepsy and food allergies are controversial at best. Several authors have proposed a possible role of food allergy in a subset of children with epilepsy [172-174]. However a great deal of additional research must be performed. Frediani et al have noted a significantly higher proportion of allergic disorders in 72 epileptic patients versus 202 aged-matched controls [173]. Using skin prick tests, the percentage of epileptic children who tested positive for cow's milk protein (24/72), lactalbumin (16/72) and β-lactoglobulin (10/72) was significantly higher than the percentage of controls who tested positive for the same allergens: 7/202 for cow's milk protein, 4/202 for lactalbumin, and 2/202 for β-lactoglobulin. In patients with allergic disorders, there is an increase in the proportion of electroencephalographic anomalies, often in the form of occipital dysrhythmias [173]. Crayton et al reported on a patient whose epileptic fits were triggered and increased in frequency by double-blind food challenges [172]. Frediani et al reported on a nine-year-old boy whose epileptic symptoms disappeared as a result of an allergen-free diet with no anticonvulsant therapy [174].

ENDOCRINE MANIFESTATION

Diabetes Mellitus

Cow's milk has been implicated as a possible trigger of an autoimmune response destroying pancreatic ß-cells in genetically susceptible individuals, thereby leading to diabetes mellitus [175-177]. Karjalainen et al measured IgG antibovine serum albumin antibodies in the serum of 142 children with newly diagnosed insulin-dependent diabetes mellitus [177]. These children had elevated serum concentrations of IgG antibovine serum albumin antibodies that declined after diagnosis and reached normal levels in most patients within one to two years. These authors speculate that patients with insulin-dependent diabetes mellitus have immunity to cow's milk albumin, with antibodies to an albumin peptide that are capable of reacting with a β-cell-specific surface protein. Such antibodies could participate in the development of islet cell dysfunction. Cavallo et al measured the in vitro peripheral T-lymphocyte response to β-casein in 47 patients with recent-onset insulin-dependent diabetes mellitus [175]. Twenty four of 47 (51.1%) patients with insulin-dependent diabetes mellitus versus 0 of 10 patients with autoimmune thyroid disease and 1 of 36 (2.8%) healthy people had a positive response to ß-casein. A positive response was defined as a stimulation index above the mean value plus 2 SD of healthy people. These authors suggest that exposure to cow's milk triggers a cellular and humoral anti- ß-casein immune response that may cross-react with a β-cell antigen and lead to destruction of the β-cell. A subsequent study, however, showed a lack of association between early exposure to cow's milk and β-cell autoimmunity [178]. Norris et al screened 253 children aged nine months to seven years with first-degree relatives who had insulin-dependent diabetes mellitus for β-cell autoimmunity [178]. Eighteen cases of β-cell autoimmunity were detected at baseline. These children were compared with 153 unrelated autoantibody-negative children selected from the cohort as controls. There were no differences in the proportion of cases and controls that were exposed to cow's milk or foods containing cow's milk by 3 months or 6 months of age. Further studies are necessary to clarity this important issue.

RENAL MANIFESTATION

Nephrotic Syndrome

Food allergy may play a role in the pathogenesis of nephrotic syndrome in a selected group of children [179-182]. Sandberg et al reported 6 children with steroid-responsive nephrotic syndrome [179]. In the relapse period, a milk-free diet led to remission without steroid therapy. In the remission period, challenge with cow's milk resulted in a relapse in 4 patients. Sieniawska et al evaluated the role of cow's milk in 17 children with steroid-resistant nephrotic syndrome [182]. Cow's milk was excluded from the diet for at least 14 days without changing the previously ineffective prednisone dosage. Six patients went into remission three to eight days after the elimination of cow's milk. After a period of two to three weeks of remission, cow's milk challenge was positive in three of the six patients. The group of responders to a milk-free diet was characterized by young age, feeding with cow's milk or unmodified powdered milk formulas in the neonatal period, and coexistence of allergic symptoms. The authors suggest that cellular mechanisms may play a role in cow's milk-induced steroid-resistant nephrotic syndrome as evidenced by the late-onset reaction to cow's milk challenge, positive leukocyte migration inhibition tests, absence of specific IgE antibodies, and negative skin test results. These studies, however, contain some design flaws and better objective studies are needed to prove the association between milk ingestion and nephrotic syndrome.

HEMATOLOGIC MANIFESTATIONS

Anemia

Iron deficiency anemia may develop in children with cow's milk allergy secondary to gastrointestinal blood loss. This may be caused by milk-induced enterocolitis syndrome, milk-induced colitis, and allergic eosinophilic gastroenteropathy, and Heiner syndrome.

Thrombocytopenia

A few anecdotal reports suggest that thrombocytopenia may be caused by food allergy [183-185]. Whitefield and Barr reported a girl with the syndrome of thrombocytopenia and absent radius who showed marked gastrointestinal disturbance with clinical evidence of cow's milk allergy and in whom there appeared to be a direct correlation between cow's milk exposure, gastro-intestinal upset, and thrombocytopenia [183]. Jones reported a newborn male infant with idiopathic thrombocytopenic purpura in whom withdrawal of a milk formula produced an improvement in the platelet count and reintroduction of the milk formula led to hematologic relapse on two occasions [184]. It has been suggested that a type II cytotoxic reaction may account for the thrombocytopenia seen after the ingestion of milk [185].

RHEUMATIC MANIFESTATIONS

Vasculitis

Food-induced vasculitis has been described [186,187]. In the majority of cases, it is mediated by type III immunologic reaction in which the antigen combines with its specific IgG and complement to form circulating complexes [186]. The circulating complexes deposit in the small blood vessels and initiate vasculitis. Occasionally, food-induced vasculitis may be IgE-mediated. Businco et al reported two patients with leucocytoclastic vasculitis confirmed by skin biopsy [186]. The first patient had cutaneous vasculitis with large joint involvement, caused by cow's milk and egg as confirmed by blind food challenge. The second patient had cutaneous and mucous membrane vasculitis with large joint involvement caused by chocolate. Lunardi et al described five patients with allergy and cutaneous vasculitis of 1 to 13 years' duration [187]. Double-blind food challenges identified the offending agent to be a food in two patients, an additive in another two patients, and both food and additive in the fifth patient.

Arthropathy/Arthritis

A few anecdotal reports suggest that arthropathy/arthritis may be the result of food hypersensitivity [188-190]. Parke et al described a 38-year-old woman who had progressive rheumatoid arthritis for 11 years [191]. Her rheumatoid arthritis improved within three weeks of changing to a milk-free diet and deteriorated within 24 hours with a milk challenge. Golding reported three patients with food-induced synovitis [192]. van de Larr et al described six patients with rheumatoid arthritis that responded to a diet limited to an elemental formula [193]. Double-blind placebo-controlled trial confirmed a relationship with specific food in four of the six patients. Long-term benefit from avoidance of the specific foods, however, was noted only in two patients. Panush monitored 97 patients with inflammatory arthritis and found that no more than 5% of the patients with rheumatic disease had immunologic sensitivity to foods [190]. Denman et al have not been able to detect any consistent correlation between controlled dietary challenges and exacerbations of inflammatory arthritis [194]. In those cases in which inflammatory arthritis responds to dietary manipulation, it is possible that dietary restriction non-specifically moderates the inflammatory manifestations of the disease or the placebo effect may be responsible [194]. Karatay et al have shown that individualized diet challenges consisting of allergenic foods may regulate tumor necrosis factor-α and interleukin-1β levels in selected patients with rheumatoid arthritis [195]. Tumor necrosis factor-α and interleukin-1β are cytokines that promote inflammation and may play an important role in the development of rheumatoid arthritis [195].

Chapter 5

CLINICAL EVALUATION
AND DIAGNOSTIC STUDIES

History and physical examination are the cornerstones for the diagnostic workup of any food allergy [6]. However, their value can fluctuate depending on dietary history recall, and timing of presentation from reaction. In this light, accurate diet diaries are invaluable tools for clinicians. Key points to document include foods consumed, route of exposure, descriptions of symptoms, timing on symptom onset and resolution, consistency of symptoms with food consumption, treatments attempted and response [5-7].

A number of diagnostic studies are indicated based on clinical impression. Several, similar diagnostic algorithms have been proposed, but no one algorithm is universally accepted [6]. Regardless, the results of these studies should be interpreted in light of history and physical examination [6]. In this light, referral to allergy specialists for testing is prudent [7]. In addition, further testing may be required to evaluate specific clinical presentations, such as endoscopy for suspected allergic eosinophilic esophagitis and biopsy for celiac disease. A detailed discussion of these numerous confirmatory tests for clinical presentations is beyond the scope of this review.

ELIMINATION DIETS

Elimination diets are frequently suggested as an initial investigation for food allergy. These diets involve the complete elimination of suspected food allergens for at least two weeks with close follow-up monitoring for resolution of clinical symptoms [6]. However, despite being fundamentally simple and cost-effective means of assessing food allergies, they are rarely diagnostic [7]. In practice, these diets are difficult to implement and require correct allergen identification, complete avoidance of the suspected allergen and the lack of other confounding factors occurring the testing period [5-7]. They are especially difficult to interpret in patients with other chronic conditions such as atopic dermatitis that may occur in isolation or as part of a constellation of symptoms with food allergy [5].

SKIN PRICK TESTING

Skin prick testing with food extracts is often used to screen patients with suspected IgE-mediated food allergies [7]. It is rapid and useful in demonstrating clinical response to allergen exposure [5]. Fundamentally, testing determines the presence of allergen-specific IgE antibodies. Patients are exposed to commercially or freshly prepared food allergens mixed with glycerin (1:10 or 1:20 ratio), as well as a positive control (generally histamine) and negative control (saline) in the form of small drops applied to the surface of the skin [5]. A "prick" is then used to break the skin barrier. By convention, a food allergen producing a wheal with a diameter 3 mm greater than the negative control is considered "positive" [5]. Because of the small risk of systemic anaphylaxis, the test should be performed in settings capable of managing this adverse event.

This test is reproducible and generally has a sensitivity of 90% but a specificity of 50% [7,196]. These values vary with age of patient, food allergen utilized. In general, commercially prepared reagents are labile and less allergenic than freshly prepared reagents with suspected fruit and vegetable allergies [6,43]. The positive predictive value and negative predictive value are 50% and 95%, respectively [197]. As such, skin prick testing is useful for ruling out IgE-mediated food allergies when results are negative, but only suggestive of possible food allergy if positive [7]. Two important exceptions include systemic anaphylaxis initiated by exposure to a single allergen which is diagnostic of food allergy and children less than one year old which may have food allergy diagnosed in the presence of a negative result [6]. Nonetheless, indiscriminate testing of multiple food allergens without clinical suspicion is not recommended as there is a fairly high potential for false positives [6].

In Vitro Tests for Total and Specific IgE

Many children with IgE-mediated food allergies have elevated serum IgE levels. Serum IgE antibodies specific for allergens can be measured in vitro by qualitative techniques such as RAST (Radio absorbant serum test), and ELISA (Enzyme-linked immunosorbant assay). In practical terms, these tests have similar sensitivity and specificity as skin-prick tests and are used in a similar fashion to screen and rule-out IgE mediated food allergies [6].

However, newer, quantitative techniques such as CAP FEIA® (Fluorenzyme immunoassay) (CAP Systems FEIA, Pharmacia-Upjohn Diagnostics) are now favored over qualitative techniques due to their greater specificity and positive predictive values [198]. Currently, for a number of foods, there are known IgE levels with a 95% positive predictive of food allergy [6]. By convention, patients with IgE levels greater than these standardized thresholds can be diagnosed with food allergy [6]. Likelihood ratio data are also available to account for varying prevalence with specific allergies in specific populations [7]. These assays are most useful when milk, egg, peanut and possibly soy, wheat and fish allergies are suspected as they are the most studied [6].

Food Challenge

An open or single-blind food challenge is practical in a clinic setting and acceptable when the resulting symptoms can be objectively observed [6]. The main disadvantage is the increased incidence of false-positive results, primarily because of biased interpretation by the patient, parents, and physician. However, the double-blind placebo-controlled food challenge has long been considered the "gold standard" for the diagnosis of food allergy. This method can be applied to both suspected IgE and non-IgE mediated food reactions [5]. This type of food challenge is objective and should be used if a positive open challenge yields only a subjective response on the part of the patient, if the symptoms are vague or ill defined, or if there is a psychological component to the reaction. However, the test can be time-consuming in a clinic setting, and carries a risk of systemic anaphylaxis and therefore is impractical for screening purposes. If IgE-mediated reactions are suspected, blinded food challenges are often initiated after a skin-prick and in vitro test has been completed. For patients being evaluated for resolution of food allergy, a food challenge will often be initiated after skin-prick and in vitro tests convert to negative.

Although no specific protocol has been widely accepted, the general principles of the food challenge are common. To begin, all foods and medications suspected of causing adverse reactions or complicating the interpretation of results are eliminated for 10 to 14 days. This allows for previous symptoms to resolve before the food challenge takes place and exaggerate any response during the food challenge [6]. The suspected food is administered in a gradual fashion, starting with a small quantity, and the dose is doubled appropriately at 15 to 20 minute intervals until symptoms occur or a reasonable serving size has been ingested. In a single blind challenge, the suspected food is hidden in some neutral, tolerated food or in capsules and the patient is unaware of the ingested food. In a double blind challenge, both the physician and patient are unaware and a neutral third party is involved. Following, patients may be observed for up to three days for symptoms, especially if a non-IgE mediated reaction is suspected [6]. Afterwards, the specific foods consumed are revealed. Extreme caution, with appropriate supports and close observation is recommended for children with previous severe systemic anaphylaxis. If the blind challenge is negative, the food should then be consumed openly in the usual quantities under observation to rule out the rare false-negative challenge.

Chapter 6

MANAGEMENT

The key to the management of food allergy is avoidance of foods known to or suspected of having caused a reaction [29]. Other approaches include pharmacotherapy, education of patients, and dietary manipulations for the prevention of food allergy in high-risk individuals. Currently, there is no effective and safe immunotherapy in the management of patients with food allergy. Referral to an allergist is generally recommended.

AVOIDANCE OF FOOD ALLERGENS

The definitive treatment of food allergy is strict elimination of the offending food from the diet [5]. It is unusual for a child to be allergic to more than one food. Bock studied 480 children with probable food hypersensitivity and found that allergic reaction to more than two foods occurred in only 10 (2.1%) of the 480 children [199]. Symptomatic reactivity to food allergens is generally very specific, and patients rarely react to more than one food in a botanical or animal species [5,49,67]. However, in pollen-related food allergy, cross-reactions can occur between phylogenetically distantly related species such as birch and kiwi or soy [200],

Although the fundamental concept is simple, avoiding an offending food antigen is often difficult in practice, especially if the offending food is ubiquitous. In particular, accidental exposure is a major obstacle. Approximately 50% of affected individuals experience accidental exposure and reactions every 3 to 5 years [201]. In addition, cross-contamination of food with the offending antigen, leading to inadvertent ingestion, is commonly described [202]. Accidents frequently occur in daycare centers, schools, and restaurants [202]. Of the 32 food-related fatalities reported by Bock et al, at least 87% of patients had a previous history of reaction to the responsible food allergen [203]. Avoidance of skin contact and inhalation of offending food allergen is also necessary [204-206].

On the other hand, the indiscriminate application of elimination diets without a firm diagnosis is a widespread malpractice and may lead to psychological dependence on an unsound diet, as well as vitamin deficiencies, malnutrition, and failure to thrive if multiple foods are inadvertently avoided [5,207-209]. Venter et al followed a birth cohort of 966 infants on the Island of Wight, United Kingdom born between September 2001 and August 2002 to the age of one year [210]. Cumulative incidence of parentally reported food hypersensitivity was 25.8%. Open or double-blind, placebo-controlled food challenges were used to confirm suspected reactions. Only 2.2% of those tested were confirmed to have food allergy, indicating the need to evaluate suspected food allergy to avoid needless dietary restriction.

In some children ingesting inappropriate elimination diets, eating disorders may develop. If elimination diets are prescribed, care must be taken to ensure that they are palatable and nutritionally adequate. Patients should be provided with information on what alternative foods are available so that good variety in the diet can be maintained [211]. A formal dietetic evaluation is recommended.

Patients and other caregivers must have a good knowledge of foods containing the allergen and must be taught to scrutinize the labels of all packaged food carefully [212]. Careful label reading is a cornerstone of food avoidance [213]. In one study, only 4 (7%) of 60 parents were able to identify milk protein in 14 sample labels [214]. Incorrect or ambiguous labeling of foods may result in accidental ingestion of the offending food [202]. Also, some of the terms used do not clearly indicate the presence of a food allergen. The United States Food and Drug Administration (FDA) now requires food manufacturers to declare and clear label all functional ingredients on food labels [215]. The Food Allergen Labeling and Consumer Protection Act (FALCPA) effective in January 2006 requires simple terms to indicate the presence of major food allergens [216]. FALCPA requires food manufacturers to state explicitly the presence of eight major food allergens, namely, milk, egg, wheat, soybean, peanut, tree nuts, fish, and shellfish. New EU labeling laws require the presence of the following food allergens at any level to be stated on the label: celery, cereals containing gluten (wheat, barley, rye and oats), crustaceans, eggs, fish, milk, mustard, tree nuts, peanuts, sesame seeds, soybeans, SO_2 and sulfites (at level >10 mg/kg or >10 mg/L) [216]. It is mandatory to list all sub-ingredients and specify the source of ingredients previously listed as "natural flavor". However, foods that are not prepackaged are not covered by this legislation [211]. Patients and/or their caregivers should be cautioned about the presence of the offending food as a "hidden" ingredient in processed foods [217,218]. In addition, at restaurants, it is important that patients learn to communicate with staff regarding their food allergies [15].

Overall, food avoidance diets in children are generally required on a transient basis as most outgrow their food allergies. As noted before, the loss of hypersensitivity is especially likely to occur in infants and young children, although older children and adults may also lose their hypersensitivity [219]. The degree of compliance with allergen avoidance and the allergen responsible may influence the outcome [220]. Consequently, rechallenge testing for food allergy should be performed; the interval between rechallenges should be dictated by the specific food allergen in question, the age of the child, and the degree of difficulty in avoiding the food in question.

ENVIRONMENTAL MANAGEMENT

Patients should be aware of high-risk environments. High-risk areas include common eating places such as childcare centers, school cafeterias, restaurants, and ice cream shops [29]. School and childcare centers should have policies facilitating food allergen avoidance such as prohibition of sharing of food or utensil and increased staff supervision during meal times [29]. Patients with reactions to airborne antigens (such as steamed fish, flour additives in Baker's asthma, peanut dust on airplanes) are at particular risk [29].

PHARMACOTHERAPY

Patients with a history of anaphylactic reaction over the age of seven years as well as caregivers should be taught how to self-administer epinephrine and should have an epinephrine autoinjector such as Anapen/Anapen Jr® (Lincoln Medical Ltd, Wiltshire, United Kingdom), EpiPen/EpiPen Jr® (Dey Pharma, L.P. of Napa, California), or Twinjet/Twinjet Jr® (Shionogi Pharma, Inc,

Georgia) and antihistamine available at all times [7,200]. It is suggested that patients at risk for anaphylaxis should always carry two doses of self-injectable epinephrine [221,222]. An identification necklace or bracelet such as MedicAlert® (MedicAlert Canada, Ontario, Canada) stating the patient's sensitivity is also advised [218]. The physician should take appropriate steps to ensure that the patients and their caregivers understand the indications and use of the device thoroughly. These individuals should also be provided with a written anaphylaxis action plan. The instructions should be clear, simple, and age appropriate. Rehearsal of the procedure is important.

Patients and/or their caregivers must be educated about early recognition of allergic symptoms and early management of an anaphylactic reaction [6]. Schools should be equipped to treat anaphylaxis in allergic students and physicians should help instruct school personnel about these issues [200]. Referral to an allergist is also recommended [223].

Epinephrine helps to block severe allergic reactions and anaphylaxis by suppressing leukotriene and histamine release [224,225]. Epinephrine reverses vasodilatation, increases blood pressure, dilates airways, reduces laryngeal edema and angioedema, and increases myocardial contractility [224,225]. For the treatment of anaphylaxis, the recommended dose of epinephrine 1:1000 (1mg/ml) is 0.01 mg/kg intramuscularly, up to a maximum of 0.3 mg (0.3 ml) in children and 0.5 mg (0.5 ml) in adults [224,226]. Peak concentrations are reached within 10 minutes of intramuscular administration [225,227]. As Anapen Jr®, EpiPen Jr®, and Twinjet Jr® contain 0.15 mg of epinephrine and Anapen®, EpiPen®, and Twinjet® contain 0.3 mg of epinephrine, it would be desirable to have a wider range of auto-injector doses [202,224]. The subcutaneous route is no longer recommended as the systemic levels of epinephrine are highly unpredictable from this mode of administration [202]. In addition intramuscular injections into the thigh result in more rapid absorption and higher plasma epinephrine levels than intramuscular injections into the arm [212,221,226,228-229]. Epinephrine works best when given early [202,224].

After first aid treatment, the patient should be transferred to the nearest emergency department for monitoring and additional treatment as required. Anaphylactic patients should continue being observed in hospital for at least 4 to 12 hours after epinephrine administration, even if they are apparently well, because of the possibility of a biphasic reaction [7]. Biphasic reactions occur in 6% of anaphylaxis with the second "peak" occurring within 4 to 12 hours in 96% of cases [7]. If necessary, epinephrine may be repeated at 5 minutes intervals [224,221]. In one study, 16% of patients presenting to the emergency department with food-induced anaphylaxis required an average of two doses of epinephrine [221].

In patients with severe anaphylaxis unresponsive to intramuscular epinephrine or with cardiovascular collapse, epinephrine should be given intravenously and transferred to intensive care with blood pressure and continuous cardiac monitoring [225,226].

Many patients also require volume support, oxygen, nebulized bronchodilators, parenteral diphenhydramine, ranitidine, and glucocorticosteroids [6,7,212,226]. Should this be the case, the patient should be placed in a recumbent position with lower limbs elevated, as tolerated symptomatically [212,226,228]. This may prevent orthostatic hypotension.

For the child with progressive or generalized urticaria or distressing pruritus, the administration of a fast-acting oral H_1 antihistamine such as hydroxyzine or diphenhydramine should be considered [67,224,226,230]. H_2 receptor blockers such as ranitidine are less helpful as only a small number of H_2 receptors are found in the skin [230]. It is critical to note that unlike epinephrine, antihistamines do not block systemic reactions in anaphylaxis [6]. They are mainly useful in relieving symptomatic pruritus [6].

The use of drugs such as disodium cromoglycate, ketotifen, and prostaglandin synthetase inhibitors in the treatment of food allergy has generally been disappointing, either because of minimal efficacy or unacceptable adverse effects [5,200]. Systemic corticosteroids are rarely used in the treatment of food allergy, except in severe anaphylaxis, allergic eosinophilic esophagitis, allergic eosinophilic gastroenteropathy, and dietary-induced enteropathy [6,231]. The side effects of long-term systemic corticosteroid therapy are unacceptable.

Currently, oral administration of activated charcoal is not considered a practical first-aid treatment for food anaphylaxis. Prophylactic medications have not been shown to be consistently effective in the prevention of severe life-threatening reactions to foods [29]. Their use may mask a less severe allergic reaction to a culprit food, the knowledge of which might prevent a more severe allergic reaction to that food in the future [29]. The use of prophylactic medications is therefore discouraged.

PROBIOTICS AND PREBIOTICS

The use of probiotics and prebiotics in the management of food allergy is controversial [232]. It has been hypothesized that the increased sensitization to food allergens might result from reduced infection or exposure to microbial products such as endotoxin in early childhood [233]. Prospective studies have found that infants who are prone to develop atopic dermatitis have lower numbers of *Bifidobacterium* in their intestinal microflora [234-236]. Evidence also suggests that probiotics may reverse the increased intestinal permeability characteristic of children with food allergy and enhance specific IgA responses frequently defective in children with food allergy [237]. *In vitro* studies show that allergic patients induce less IL-10 production and more proinflammatory cytokine production than those nonallergic individuals [238,239]. Presumably, probiotics act on the intestinal mucosa and stimulate T-cell differentiation in favor of Th1 over Th2, with resultant decreased production of IgE and increased production of IgA [238,240]. Probiotics might also correct aberrations in gut permeability [241,242]. Prebiotics work by selectively stimulating the growth or activity of a limited number of bacterial strains in the intestinal flora.

Much work has been done on the use of probiotics and, to a lesser extent, prebiotics in the management of atopic dermatitis. Several randomized controlled trials failed to show the beneficial effects of probiotics in the prevention of atopic dermatitis [243]. Other studies yielded different results [243-248]. Kalliomäki et al randomized 159 mothers and their respective infants with a family history of atopy to receive either a placebo or 10^{10} CFU of *Lactobacillus* GG for 2 to 4 weeks before delivery and for 6 months after delivery, respectively [244]. Twenty three percent of the children in the probiotic group versus 46% of children in the control group were found to have atopic dermatitis at two years of age (RR: 0.51; 95% confidence interval: 0.32-0.84) [244]. The effect was still observed two years later: 26% of children in the treatment group versus 46% of children in the placebo group had atopic dermatitis (RR: 0.57; 95% confidence interval: 0.33-0.97) [245].

Viljanen et al randomized 230 infants who had suspected cow's milk allergy in a double-blinded study to receive *L. rhamnosus* GG (n=80), a mixture of four probiotic strains (n=76), or a placebo (n=74), given twice daily with food for four weeks [248]. The authors found that *L. rhamnosus* GG was an effective therapy for atopic dermatitis in IgE-sensitized infants but not in non-IgE-sensitized infants.

In a double-blind, placebo-controlled trial, Tamura et al randomized 109 adult patients with allergic rhinitis to drink fermented milk containing *Lactobacilli casei* strain Shirota (n=55) or placebo (n=54) for 8 weeks [249]. The authors found no significant difference between the two groups during the ingestion period. In the subgroup of patients with moderate to severe nasal symptom scores before starting ingestion of test samples, supplementation with the probiotic tended to reduce nasal symptom-medication scores.

In a double-blind placebo-controlled trial, Taylor et al randomized 226 newborn infants of atopic mothers to receive either 3 x 10^9 CFU of *Lactobacillus acidophilus* (n=115) or placebo (n=111) daily for 6 months [250]. A total of 178 infants (89 in each group) completed the study. The authors found that the rates of atopic dermatitis were similar in the two groups at 6 months and 12 months of follow-up. At 12 months, the rate of sensitization was significantly higher in the probiotic group (p=0.03). These findings challenge the use of probiotics in the prevention of allergy.

Kukkonen et al randomized 1,223 pregnant women carrying high risk infants at increased risk for allergy to receive a probiotic (n=610) or a placebo (n=613) for 2 to 4 weeks before delivery [251]. Their infants received the same probiotic plus galacto-oligosaccharides (n=461) or a placebo (n=464) for 6 months. These children were evaluated at 2 years of age for cumulative incidence of allergic diseases (food allergy, eczema, asthma, and allergic rhinitis) and IgE sensitization (positive skin prick test response or serum antigen-specific IgE level). The authors found that probiotic and prebiotic treatment, compared with placebo, had no effect on the cumulative incidence of allergic diseases but tended to reduce IgE-associated atopic diseases (odds ratio: 0.71; 95% confidence interval: 0.5 to 1; p=0.052). Probiotic and prebiotic treatment did reduce eczema (odds ratio: 0.74; 95% confidence interval: 0.55 to 0.98; p=0.35) and atopic eczema (odds ratio: 0.66; 95% confidence interval: 0.46 to 0.95; p=0.025).

In a double-blind placebo-controlled trial, Weston et al randomized 56 children aged 6 to 18 months who had moderate to severe atopic dermatitis to receive *L. fementum* VRI-033 PCC (n=28) or placebo (n=28) twice daily for eight weeks [252]. Fifty children completed the study. The authors found that the reduction in the SCORAD index was significant in the probiotic group (p=0.03) but not in the placebo group. In a double-blind study, Passeron et al randomized 48 children to receive either *L. rhamnosus* Lcr 35 plus a prebiotic preparation (n=28) or an identically appearing probiotic preparation alone three times a day for three months [253]. In the symbiotic group, the mean total SCORAD score was 39.1 before treatment versus 20.7 after three months of treatment (p< 0.0001). In the probiotic group, the mean SCORAD score was 39.3 before treatment versus 24 after three months of treatment (p<0.0001). The authors concluded that symbiotics and prebiotics used alone were effective in the treatment of atopic dermatitis.

Probiotics and prebiotics are included in some infant formulas with the aim of inducing the development of a *Bifidobacterium*-dominated intestinal flora. At present, probiotics or prebiotics are not established treatment modalities for atopic dermatitis [232,238]. They are ineffective in the prevention and treatment of reactive airway disease [238]. The routine use of probiotics and prebiotics in food allergy management requires further study

DIETARY MANIPULATION IN THE PREVENTION OF FOOD ALLERGY IN THE GENERAL POPULATION

Recently, perspectives on dietary manipulation and food allergies have dramatically changed. According to a recent landmark clinical report (intended to replace previous position statements) by the Committee on Nutrition and Section on Allergy and Immunology of the American Academy of Pediatrics, there is now limited evidence to support dietary manipulation in preventing food allergies in the general, low-risk population [254].

Although evidence for prevention of atopic dermatitis and wheezing in early life is conflicting, there is insufficient evidence that exclusively breastfeeding prevents food allergy [7,254]. Long-term, randomized, control trials have shown no significant difference in risk of food allergy at 7-years of age in children exclusively breastfed from mothers on allergen-elimination diets [255, 256]. Nonetheless, breastfeeding is still recommended for its other well-described benefits in children.

Furthermore, because small amounts of food antigens ingested by the mother are excreted in breast milk [219], previous position statements by the AAP recommended avoidance of allergenic foods by lactating mothers [217,257,258]. However, this theoretical risk has not been observed. As summarized in a Cochrane review, there is inefficient evidence supporting maternal avoidance of common food allergens during breastfeeding in order to prevent food allergies in their children [254,259]. Currently, no specific dietary modification is recommended by lactating mothers. This position represents a change from previous statements.

Perhaps most dramatic, is the controversial shift in perspective with tapered introduction of solid foods to a child's diet. Traditionally, it was believed that the delayed introduction of common food allergens such as dairy, eggs, peanuts and tree nuts past 6 months chronological age would prevent food allergies [7]. However, despite being adopted into widespread clinical practice, there is little clinical evidence to support the efficacy of delayed solid introduction in preventing food allergies. In a recent major prospective birth cohort study (n=2073) by the Influences of Lifestyle-Related Factors on the Immune System and the Development of Allergies in Childhood (LISA) study group, no evidence was found to support the delayed introduction of solids in preventing food allergy [260]. In fact, some studies have shown that delayed introduction of food allergens actually confers a higher risk for future food allergy [261,262]. Given these findings, a joint-consensus document by the Adverse Reactions to Foods Committee, American College of Allergy, Asthma and Immunology currently states that the introduction of solids into an infant's diet should be individualized, and that egg, peanut, tree nuts, fish and seafood may be introduced, with caution, at six months age [263]. The American Academy of Pediatrics's recent clinical report acknowledges this lack of evidence but does not comment on clinical practice recommendations [254].

It has been suggested that supplementation with long-chain poly-unsaturated fatty acids might reduce the incidence of atopic diseases [264-266]. A Cochrane systematic review showed no consistent beneficial effect on marine fatty acids (fish oil) supplementation in asthma prevention [267]. A meta-analysis showed that supplementation with fish oil did not improve the severity of atopic dermatitis [268].

DIETARY MANIPULATION IN THE PREVENTION OF FOOD ALLERGY IN HIGH-RISK INDIVIDUALS

Evidence supporting the reduction of food allergy by dietary manipulation mainly applies to high-risk populations, defined by the American Academy of Pediatrics as infants with at least one first-degree relative with allergic disease [254]. Consequently, recommendations in high-risk individuals remain largely unchanged from previous position statements [254].

In high-risk infants, there is limited evidence that exclusive breastfeeding and delaying of solids until six months of age, breastfeeding might delay, or possibly prevent, the onset of food allergy [269]. A number of potential mechanisms have been proposed for the potential protective effects of breastfeeding. Colostrum may provide a protective coating to the gut that prevents the entrance of large foreign proteins and minimizing the possibility of an allergic response. Breastfeeding reduces the amount of foreign protein in the gastrointestinal tract and passively transfers maternal IgA to the infant, which minimizes the risk for absorption of antigens from the gastrointestinal tract. Transfer of cell-mediated immunity from mother to infant stimulates IgA synthesis in the infant [257]. Epidermal growth factor present in human milk hastens maturation of intestinal mucosa and epithelium, and strengthens the mucosal barrier to antigen. Several studies have shown that respiratory and gastrointestinal infections can predispose to the development of allergic diseases [257]. The allergy-preventive effect of breastfeeding might be secondary to a reduction in the number of infections in the infant.

Although evidence for food allergies is limited, partially hydrolysed formulas are often used for the prevention of atopy when breastfeeding is not possible in infants with a strong family history of allergy or elevated cord IgE levels to reduce possible food allergy symptoms [270]. These formulas have been developed with the aim of minimizing the number of sensitizing epitopes within milk proteins, while at the same time retaining peptides of sufficient size and immunogenicity to stimulate the induction of oral tolerance. Compared with extensively hydrolysed formulas, partially hydrolysed formulas are less expensive and more palatable [220]. Prospective controlled trials examining the use of extensively hydrolysed formulas and partially hydrolysed formulas for allergy prevention among high-risk infants show significant reductions in the cumulative incidence of atopic disease through the first five years of life compared with those fed with cow's milk formulas [270]. In the meta-analysis performed by Osborn et al, infants fed extensively hydrolysed formulas versus partially hydrolysed formulas had a significant reduction in food allergy (two studies, 341 infants; typical risk ratio: 0.43; 95%confidence interval: 0.19 to 0.99), but there was no significant difference in all allergy or any other specific allergy incidence [122].

Soy protein is immunogenic and allergenic, although less than cow's milk [272]. A meta-analysis of two studies (n=283) found no significant differences in childhood allergy cumulative incidence from the use of a soy formula compared to a cow's milk formula (typical risk ratio: 0.67; 95% confidence interval: 0.18 to 2.46) [273]. As there is no evidence of benefit, the use of a soy formula for prevention of food allergy cannot be recommended [254,273,274].

There is also evidence suggesting that early introduction of solid food may increase the risk of food allergy in high-risk individuals [274-277]. The existing literature suggests that the optimal developmental time for the introduction of selected supplemental food should be six months. For infants at risk, dairy products should not be introduced before 12 months, eggs 24 months, and peanut, tree nuts, fish, and seafood at least 36 months of age [278]. It is recommended that foods should be introduced one at a time and gradually [278]. Cooked, homogenized foods should be preferred to their fresh counterparts when a reduction of allergenicity has been clinically demonstrated for that processed food [278].

Marini et al prospectively studied 279 infants with high atopic risk who were put on an allergy prevention program and 80 infants with similar atopic risk but no intervention [279]. The intervention program included dietary measures (exclusive and prolonged milk feeding followed by a hypoallergenic weaning diet) and environmental measures such as avoidance of parental smoking in the presence of the babies. The incidence of allergic manifestations was much lower in the intervention group than in the nonintervention group at 1 year (11.5% vs. 54.4%), 2 years (14.9% vs. 65.6%), and 3 years (20.6% vs. 74.1%). Atopic dermatitis and recurrent wheezing were found in both the intervention group and the nonintervention group from birth to the second year of life, whereas urticaria and gastrointestinal disorders were only present in the nonintervention group in the first year of life. Halken et al studied 105 "high-risk" infants who were breast-fed and/or receiving a hypoallergenic formula combined with avoidance of solid foods during the first 6 months of life [280]. This prevention group was compared with a control group consisting of 54 identically defined "high-risk" infants who were on an unrestricted diet. The cumulative prevalence of atopic symptoms was significantly lower at 18 months in the prevention group (32%) than in the control group (74%) (p < 0.01) because of a reduced prevalence of recurrent wheezing (13% vs. 37%; p < 0.01), atopic dermatitis (14% vs. 31%; p < 0.01), vomiting/diarrhea (5% vs. 28%; p < 0.01), and infantile colic (9% vs. 24%; p < 0.01). The cumulative prevalence of food allergy was significantly lower in the prevention group (6% vs. 17%; p < 0.05). The authors concluded that feeding high-risk infants with breast milk and/or hypoallergenic formula, combined with the avoidance of solid foods during the first 6 months of life, has a protective effect on the risk of atopic dermatitis developing during the first 18 months of life.

MISCELLANEOUS ASPECTS

Infants with cow's milk protein allergy should avoid cow's milk or formulas containing intact cow's milk proteins [281]. It has been estimated that 15 to 25% of infants who have IgE-mediated cow's milk allergy are also allergic to soy, but the rate of tolerance is only 50% for those with non-IgE-mediated cow's milk allergy [45,282]. Soy proteins have been identified that cross-react with cow's milk caseins [283]. A Cochrane analysis of studies comparing soy to hydrolysed cow's milk formulas found no significant difference in infant and childhood allergy and atopic disease [273]. As such, soy formula is not recommended for the prevention of allergy, or for food intolerance [284]. In addition, goat's milk is not recommended in infants with cow's milk allergy as goat's milk also shares some allergenic protein fractions with cow's milk [284,285]. Infants with cow's milk or soy hypersensitivity should be fed a hypoallergenic formula [286]. Extensively hydrolysed casein formulas such as Nutramigen® (Mead Johnson Nutrition [Canada] Co., Ottawa, Canada), Pregestimil® (Mead Johnson Nutrition [Canada] Co., Ottawa, Canada), and Alimentum® (Abbott Laboratories, Limited, Saint-Laurent, Quebec, Canada) have also been used successfully in this regard [286,287]. These formulas are hypoallergenic and well tolerated by children [288]. These formulas, however, are expensive and unpalatable. The partially hydrolyzed whey hydrolysate formulas such as Good Start® (Nestle Canada, Ontario, Canada) is less expensive and have a better taste [220]. However, it contains slightly larger peptides and significantly more immunologically identifiable cow's milk protein, and therefore not suitable for the treatment of cow's milk allergy [283]. Formulas whose protein source is free amino acids are available and are considered as nonallergenic. These formulas should be tried in infants who are very sensitive to cow's milk protein and cannot tolerate even extensively hydrolysed formulas. However, they are also very expensive. Amino acid-based formulas are also useful in the treatment of allergic eosinophilic esophagitis and allergic eosinophilic gastroenteropathy [289-291].

Patients with oral allergy syndrome generally do not experience symptoms when their offending fruit or vegetable is cooked, as proteinacious antigens are generally denatured by heat [35]. Thus, patients with this presentation can consumed cooked food antigen, but should avoid uncooked food antigens.

Chapter 7

FUTURE THERAPEUTIC OPTIONS

There is currently no effective and safe specific immunotherapy for food allergens. The study of injectable specific immune therapy using peanuts was suspended because of the high rate of adverse reactions [292]. Traditional injection immunotherapy for other food allergies is not recommended either because of the risk of serious systemic reactions associated with such therapy [293]. Sublingual immunotherapy to food allergens is better tolerated and preliminary results are encouraging [289,294,295]. Long-term efficiency of sublingual immunotherapy, however, remains to be determined.

Vaccines for immunotherapy specially for food-induced anaphylaxis that are being developed include humanized anti-IgE monoclonal antibody therapy, sublingual immunotherapy, peptide immunotherapy, mutated protein immunotherapy, plasmid DNA immunotherapy, engineered recombinant protein immunotherapy, immunostimulatory sequence-modulated immune-therapy, cytokine-modulated immunotherapy, bacterial-encapsulated allergen immunotherapy, and homologous protein immunotherapy [5,202,295-298]. Allergen-specific immunotherapy should be considered for patients who have specific IgE antibodies to clinically relevant allergens and whose allergic symptoms are severe enough to warrant the time and risk of allergen immunotherapy [295].

Preliminary studies showed the potential use of humanized monoclonal anti-IgE antibody in food-allergic subjects [299,300]. Humanized monoclonal anti-IgE antibody binds to the third domain of the Fc region of the IgE molecule and prevents its binding to the high affinity receptor on mast cells and basophils [301]. The anti-IgE also down regulates the expression of the high affinity receptor on mast cells and decreases the release of histamine from phils [302]. In a randomized, double-blind, placebo-controlled trial in 84 patients with a history of peanut allergy, Leung et al showed an increased threshold of tolerance in patients with severe peanut allergy on oral food challenge after being given every 4 weeks subcutaneous injection of TNX-901 for four doses [296]. TNX-901 is a humanized IgG_1 monoclonal antibody against IgE that binds with high affinity to an epitope in the CH_3 domain [296]. The effect was highly significant at the 450 mg dose level. However, even at the highest dose of TNX-901, approximately 25% of patients were not protected. The treatment was well tolerated with no systemic adverse events. Unfortunately, anti-IgE therapy is expensive and such therapy has to be administered on a regular basis so as to maintain its protective effect [6,15]. Currently, another anti-IgE humanized IgG_1 antibody (omalizumab) is being tested in subjects older than 6 years of age with peanut anaphylaxis [206]. Stern et al treated four adults with eosinophilic esophagitis with a human monoclonal IgG_1 antibody against interleukin-5 (mepolizumab) given by infusion on a monthly basis [303]. After three months of treatment (750 mg monthly), the mean and maximal esophageal eosinophilic count fell from 46 to 6 and from 153 to 28 per high-power field, respectively. The patients also reported improvement of clinical symptoms and quality of life.

Oral immunotherapy seems to represent an interesting and promising approach for the management of food allergy [295]. Enrique et al randomized in a double-blind, placebo-controlled fashion 23 patients with hazelnut allergy to receive either a standardized hazelnut extract or placebo using a sublingual-spit rush protocol over four days [304]. They then received maintenance sublingual immunotherapy for approximately three months. On repeat double-blind, placebo-controlled food challenge, patients in the treatment group had a mean quantity of hazelnut provoking objective symptoms and increased tolerance to hazelnuts from 2.29 gm to 11.59 gm (p=0.02) while patients in the placebo group had a non-significant increase from 3.49 gm to 4.14 gm.

Peptide immunotherapy utilizes peptide fragments containing T-cell-reactive epitopes rather complete protein molecules [293]. Apparently, this kind of therapy would induce T-cell unresponsiveness and production of interferon-γ in a concentration-dependent manner [206]. Peptide immunotherapy allows for formulation of vaccines against any target in which major allergenic proteins are known because IgE binding sites for each major allergen do not have to be mapped [206]. It is hoped that such therapy would render T-cells unresponsive to subsequent allergen exposure. Peptide immunotherapy might play a role in the future therapy of food allergy.

Mutated protein immunotherapy is based on the modification of the primary amino acid sequences of IgE-binding allergenic epitopes of the major allergens present in food, with the aim of reducing allergen potential thereby eliminating activation of mast cells and basophils [206,293]. Mutation of the IgE-binding sites leaves the T-cell response unaffected [305]. The large numbers of allergens present in each food hampers such therapy.

Plasmid DNA immunotherapy results in transcription and translation of encoded genes and elicits an antibody response in the host, thereby preferentially induces a Th1 immune response and suppression of IgE [201,306] Plasmid DNA requires immunostimulatory sequences for optimal immunogenicity [306].

Engineered recombinant protein technology makes room for the development of hypoallergenic derivatives of natural allergens, which would minimize the adverse effect of immunotherapy. Such allergens should not be able to activate cells via cross-linking of IgE antibodies, but should preserve T-cell epitopes and activate B-cells to induce blocking IgG antibodies [201].

Immunostimulatory sequence-modulated immunotherapy using CpG has been shown to be effective in reversing IgE-mediated sensitization in patients with ragweed allergy [307,308]. Likewise, immunostimulatory sequence-conjugated Ara h 2 has been shown to be beneficial in the treatment allergy in a murine model [6].

In animal studies, various Chinese herbs have been shown to block anaphylactic reactions resulting from food allergy [309-311]. The therapeutic effect was associated with immunoregulatory effects on Th1-Th-2 responses and reductions in IgE levels [310]. The exact mechanism is not known and further studies are required.

Chapter 8

VACCINATIONS AND FOOD ALLERGIES

Although measles-German measles-mumps (MMR) vaccine is cultured from chick embryos, MMR vaccination is not contraindicated in children allergic to eggs [224,312]. The vaccine should, however, be administered in a supervised setting. On the other hand, the vaccine is contraindicated in children with known systemic allergic reaction to neomycin or gelatin as most reported drug allergies are due to these vaccine components [313].

According to the American Academy of Pediatrics, the influenza and yellow fever vaccines, which are cultured in chick embryo and contain small amounts of egg protein, should be avoided in those with severe anaphylactic reactions [314]. For those with non-anaphylactoid reactions, skin prick testing with the vaccine should be performed. Those with positive results should receive their vaccine in divided graded doses with close supervision after administration [314]. The recommended schedule is 0.05 ml of 1:10 dilution, followed by 0.05 mL, 0.10 mL, 0.15 mL and 0.20 mL of full strength vaccine, with doses spaced 15 to 20 minutes apart [314].

Chapter 9

CONCLUSION

Food allergy is an inappropriate immunological response to exposed food. This immunological response is primarily IgE-mediated, but can also occur through other, non-IgE-mediated mechanisms. Food allergy primarily affects infants, with a natural history tending towards resolution by adulthood. In recent years, food allergy has clearly been shown to be increasing in prevalence. Although much remains unknown about this phenomenon, recent studies regarding the precise pathogenic mechanisms have begun to shed light on the matter.

Clinically, food allergy can present in an extraordinarily diverse manner. Typically, food allergy affects multiple organs, with the gastrointestinal, dermatological/integument and respiratory systems most commonly involved. Given this diversity, there is often a tendency for patients to over-report food allergy. Hence diagnosis can be a challenge. Skin prick tests, as well as in vitro testing have been applied with success for screening, but the gold standard for diagnosis remains a double blinded placebo control food trial. The slightly more practical, single blinded placebo controlled food trial can also be administered under the right circumstances.

Of the various clinical presentations of food allergy, systemic anaphylaxis is potentially the most important to recognize as it is potentially fatal and requires immediate management. Prompt airway management and intramuscular epinephrine injection are the cornerstones of management. In terms of long-term management, allergenic avoidance remains the mainstay of therapy, although other interventions such as dietary modification to prevent food allergy have been attempted with mixed results. In recent years, policies on dietary modification to prevent food allergy have changed considerably, with modification now recommended for those with higher risk of food allergy, rather than the general population as previously suggested. Therapies on the horizon include vaccination and immunotherapy.

REFERENCES

[1] Leung, AK. Food allergy: a clinical approach. *Adv. Pediatr.* 1998;45:145-177.

[2] Leung, AK; Kamat, D. Clinical manifestations of food allergy. In: Chesterton, CM, (ed). *Food Allergies: New Research.* New York: Nova Science Publishers, Inc., 2008, pp.91-120.

[3] Leung, AK; Hon, KL. Management of the child with food allergy. In: Chesterton CM, (ed). *Food Allergies: New Research.* New York: Nova Science Publishers, Inc., 2008, pp.135-156.

[4] Burks, W; Ballmer-Weber, BK. Food allergy. *Mol. Nutr. Food Res.* 2006;50:595-603.

[5] Scurlock, AM; Lee, LA; Burks, AW. Food allergy in children. *Immunol. Allergy Clin. North Am.* 2005;25:369-388.

[6] Sampson, HA. Update on food allergy. *J. Allergy Clin. Immunol.* 2004;113:805-819.

[7] Lack, G. Food allergy. *N. Engl. J. Med.* 2008;359:1252-1260.

[8] Thong, BY; Hourihane, JO. Monitoring of IgE-mediated food allergy in childhood. *Acta Paediatr.* 2004;93:759-764.

[9] Bock, SA. Prospective appraisal of complaints of adverse reactions to foods in children during the first 3 years of life. *Pediatrics.* 1987;79: 683-688.

[10] Skolnick, HS; Conover-Walker, MK; Koerner, CB; et al. The natural history of peanut allergy. *J. Allergy Clin. Immunol.* 2001;107:367-374

[11] Cocharane, S; Beyer, K; Clausen, M; et al. Factor influencing the incidence and prevalence of food allergy. *Allergy.* 2009;64:1246-1255.

[12]   Grundy, J; Bateman, BJ; Gantm, C; et al. Peanut allergy in three year old children - a population based study. *J. Allergy Clin. Immunol.* 2001;107(suppl):S231.

[13]   Sicherer, SH; Munoz-Furlong, A; Sampson, HA. Prevalence of peanut and tree nut allergy in the United States determined by means of a random digit dial telephone survey: a 5-year follow-up study. *J. Allergy Clin. Immunol.* 2003;112:1203-1207.

[14]   Asero, R; Ballmer-Weber, BK; Beyer, K; et al. IgE-mediated food allergy diagnosis: current status and new perspectives. *Mol. Nutr. Food Res.* 2007;51:135-147.

[15]   Keet, CA; Wood RA. Food allergy and anaphylaxis. *Immunol. Allergy Clin. North Am.* 2007;27:193-212.

[16]   Jyonouchi H. Non-IgE medited food allergy. *Inflamm. Allergy Drug Targets.* 2008;7(3):173-180.

[17]   Sampson, HA. The immunopathogenic role of food hypersensitivity in atopic dermatitis. *Acta Derm. Venereol.* 1992;176:S34-S37.

[18]   Golbert, TM; Patterson, R; Pruzansky, JJ. Systemic allergic reactions to ingested antigens. *J. Allergy.* 1969;44:96-107.

[19]   Joint Task Force on Practice Parameters; American Academy of Allergy, Asthma and Immunology; American College of Allergy, Asthma and Immunology; Joint Council of Allergy, Asthma and Immunology. The diagnosis and management of anaphylaxis: an updated practice parameter. *J. Allergy Clin. Immunol.* 2005;115:S483-S523.

[20]   Sampson, HA. Anaphylaxis and emergency treatment. *Pediatrics.* 2003;111: 1601-1608.

[21]   Brigino, E; Bahna, SL. Clinical features of food allergy in infants. *Clin. Rev. Allergy Immunol.* 1995;13:329-345.

[22]   Brown, SG. Cardiovascular aspects of anaphylaxis: implications for treatment and diagnosis. *Curr. Opin. Allergy Clin. Immunol.* 2005;5:359-364.

[23]   Anderson, JA. Food allergy and intolerance. In: Lieberman, P; Anderson, JA. (eds). *Current Clinical Practice: Allergic Diseases: Diagnosis and Treatment.* 3rd edition. Totowa: Humana Press, 2007, pp. 271-294.

[24]   Wang, J; Sampson, HA. Food anaphylaxis. *Clin. Exp. Allergy.* 2007;37:651-660.

[25]   Maulitz, RM; Pratt, DS; Schocket, AL. Exercise-induced anaphylactic reactions to shellfish. *J. Allergy Clin. Immunol.* 1979;63:433-434.

[26] Sheffer, AL; Austen, KF. Exercise-induced anaphylaxis. *J. Allergy Clin. Immunol.* 1980;66:106-111.

[27] Kidd, JM III; Cohen, SH; Sosman, AJ; et al. Food-dependent exercise-induced anaphylaxis. *J. Allergy Clin. Immunol.* 1983;71:407-411.

[28] Beaudouin, E; Renaudin, JM; Morisset, M; et al. Food-dependent exercise-induced anaphylaxis – update and current data. *Eur. Ann. Allergy Clin. Immunol.* 2006;38:45-51.

[29] American College of Allergy, Asthma, & Immunology. Food allergy: a practice parameter. *Ann. Allergy Asthma Immunol.* 2006;96(Suppl 2):S1-S68.

[30] Noma, T; Yoshizawa, I; Ogawa, N; et al. Fatal buckwheat dependent exercise induced anaphylaxis. *Asian Pacific J. Allergy Immunol.* 2001;19:283-286.

[31] Dohi, M; Suko, M; Sugiyama, H; et al. 3 cases of food-dependent exercise-induced anaphylaxis in which aspirin intake exacerbated anaphylactic symptoms. *Arerugi.* 1990;39:1598-1604.

[32] Morita, E; Kunie, K; Matsuo, H. Food-dependent exercise-induced anaphylaxis. *J. Dermatol. Sci.* 2007;47:109-117.

[33] Anderson, JA. The clinical spectrum of food allergy in adults. *Clin. Exp. Allergy.* 1991;21:S304-S315.

[34] Silverstein, SR; Frommer, DA; Dobozin, B; et al. Celery-dependent exercise-induced anaphylaxis. *J. Emerg. Med.* 1986;4:195-199.

[35] Nash, S; Burks, AW. Oral allergy syndrome. *Curr. Allergy Asthma Rep.* 2007;7:1-2.

[36] Sugita, K; Kabashima, K; Nakashima, D; et al. Oral allergy syndrome caused by raw fish in a Japanese sushi bar worker. *Contact dermatitis.* 2007;56:369-370.

[37] Purohit-Sheth, TS; Carr, WW. Oral allergy syndrome (pollen-food allergy syndrome). *Allergy Asthma Proc.* 2005;26:229-230.

[38] Seidman, E. Food allergic disorders of the gastrointestinal tract. In: Roy, CC; Silverman, A; Allagille, D. (eds). *Pediatric Clinical Gastroenterology.* St Louis: Mosby. 1995; pp. 374-384.

[39] Sampson, HA. Food allergy – accurately identifying clinical reactivity. *Allergy.* 2005;60:19-24.

[40] Aiuti, F ; Paganelli, R. Food allergy and gastrointestinal diseases. *Ann. Allergy.* 1983;51:275-280.

[41] Amlot, PL; Kemeny, DM; Zachary, C; et al. Oral allergy syndrome: symptoms of IgE mediated hypersensitivity to foods. *Clin. Allergy.* 1987;17:33-42.

[42]   Lee, LA; Buirks, AW. Food allergies: prevalence, molecular characterization, and treatment/prevention strategies. *Annu. Rev. Nutr.* 2006;26;539-565.

[43]   Ortolani, C; Ispano, M; Pastorello, EA; et al. Comparison of results of skin prick tests (with fresh foods and commercial food extracts) and RAST in 100 patients with oral allergy syndrome. *J. Allergy Clin. Immunol.* 1989;83:683-690.

[44]   Hallett, R; Teuber, SS. Food allergies and sensitivities. *Nutr. Clin. Care.* 2004;7:122-129.

[45]   Garcia-Careaga, M; Kerner, JA, Jr. Gastrointestinal manifestations of food allergies in pediatric patients. *Nutr. Clin. Pract.* 2005;20:526-535.

[46]   Spergel, JM; Pawlowski, NA. Food allergy: mechanisms, diagnosis, and management in children. *Pediatr. Clin. North Am.* 2002;49:73-96.

[47]   Strobel, S; Hourihane, OB. Gastrointestinal allergy: clinical symptoms and immunological mechanisms. *Pediatr. Allergy Immunol.* 2001;12(Suppl 14):43-46.

[48]   Pastorello, EA; Robino, AM. Clinical role of lipid transfer proteins in food allergy. *Mol. Nutr. Food Res.* 2004;48:356-362.

[49]   Hoffman, KM; Sampson, HA. Evaluation and management of patients with adverse food reactions. In: Bierman, CW; Pearlman, DS; Shapiro, GG; et al. (eds). *Allergy, Asthma, and Immunology from Infancy to Adulthood.* Philadelphia: WB Saunders. 1996; pp. 665-686.

[50]   Sicherer, SH. Clinical aspects of gastrointestinal food allergy in childhood. *Pediatrics.* 2003;111:1609-1616.

[51]   Dauer, EH; Freese, DK; El-Youssef, M; et al. Clinical characteristics of eosinophilic esophagitis in children. *Ann. Otol. Rhinol. Laryngol.* 2005;114:827-833.

[52]   Furuta, GT; Straumann, A. Review article: the pathogensis and management of eosinophilic oesophagitis. *Aliment. Pharmacol. Ther.* 2006;24:173-182.

[53]   Heine, RG. Pathophysiology, diagnosis and treatment of food protein-induced gastrointestinal diseases. *Curr. Opin. Allergy Clin. Immunol.* 2004;4:221-229.

[54]   Spergel, JM. Eosinophilic esophagitis in adults and children: evidence for a food allergy component in many patients. *Curr. Opin. Allergy Clin. Immunol.* 2007;7:274-278.

[55]   Furuta, T; Liacouras CA; Collins, MH; et al. Eosinophilic esophagitis in children and adults: a systemic review and consensus recommendations for diagnosis and treatment. *Gastroenterology.* 2007;133:1342-1363.

[56]   Noel, RJ; Rothenberg, ME. Eosinophilic esophagitis. *Curr. Opin. Pediatr.* 2005;17:690-694.

[57]   Martin-Muñoz, MF; Lucendo, AJ; Navarro, M, et al. Food allergies and eosinophilic esophagitis – two case studies. *Digestion.* 2006;74:49-54

[58]   Pentiuk, SP; Miller, CK; Kaul, A. Eosinophilic esophagitis in infants and toddlers. *Dysphagia.* 2007;22:44-48.

[59]   Cheung, KM; Oliver, MR; Cameron, DJ, et al. Esophageal eosinophilia in children with dysphagia. *J. Pediatr. Gastroenterol. Nutr.* 2003;37:498-503.

[60]   Croese, J; Fairley, SK; Masson, JW; et al. Clinical and endoscopic features of eosinophilic esophagitis in adults. *Gastrointest. Endosc.* 2003;58:516-522.

[61]   Liacouras, CA. Eosinophilic esophagitis in children and adults. *J. Pediatr. Gastroenterol. Nutr.* 2003;37:S23-S28.

[62]   Kaczmarski, SJ. Gastroesophageal reflux in children and adolescents. Clinical aspects with special respect to food hypersensitivity. *Adv. Med. Sci.* 2006;51:327-335.

[63]   Kelly, KJ; Lazenby, AJ; Rowe, PC; et al. Eosinophilic esophagitis attributed to gastroesophageal reflux: improvement with an amino acid-based formula. *Gastroenterology.* 1995;109:1503-1512.

[64]   Gonsalves, N. Food allergies and eosinophilic gastrointestinal illness. *Gastroenterol. Clin. North Am.* 2007;36:75-91.

[65]   Klein, NC; Hargrove, RI; Sleisenger, MH; et al. Eosinophilic gastroenteritis. *Medicine (Baltimore).* 1970;49:299-319

[66]   Proujansky, R; Winter, HS; Walker, WA. Gastrointestinal syndromes associated with food sensitivity. *Adv. Pediatr.* 1988;35:219-238.

[67]   Bock, SA; Sampson, HA. Food allergy in infancy. *Pediatr. Clin. North Am.* 1994;41:1047-1067.

[68]   Mansueto, P; Montalto, G; Pacor, ML; et al. Food allergy in gastroenterologic diseases: review of literature. *World J. Gastroenterol.* 2006;12:7744-7752.

[69]   Pirson, F. Food allergy: a challenge for the clinician. *Acta Gastroenterol. Belg.* 2006;69:38-42.

[70]   Nowak-Wegrzyn, A; Sampson, HA; Wood, RA; et al. Food protein-induced enterocolitis syndrome caused by solid food proteins. *Pediatrics.* 2003;111:829-835.

[71]   Murch, S. Allergy and intestinal dysmotility – evidence of genuine causal linkage? *Curr. Opin. Gastroenterol.* 2006;22:664-668.

[72]   Yimyaem, P; Chongsrisawat, V; Vivatvakin, B, et al. Gastrointestinal manifestations of cow's milk protein allergy during the first year of life. *J. Med. Assoc. Thai.* 2003;86:116-123.

[73]   Hojsak, I; Kljaić-Turkalj, M; Mišak. Z; et al. Rice protein-induced enterocolitis syndrome. *Clin. Nutr.* 2006;25:533-536.

[74]   Sampson, HA. Food allergies. In: Oski, FA; DeAngelis, CD; Feigin, RD. (eds). *Principles and Practice of Pediatrics.* Philadelphia: JB Lippincott. 1994; pp. 227-232.

[75]   Lake, AM. Dietary protein enterocolitis. *Curr. Allergy Rep.* 2001;1:76-79.

[76]   Hirose, R; Yamada, T; Hayashida, Y. Massive bloody stools in two neonates caused by cow's milk allergy. *Pediatr. Surg. Int.* 2006;22:935-938.

[77]   Swart, JF; Ultee, K. Rectal bleeding in a preterm infant as a symptom of allergic colitis. *Eur. J. Pediatr.* 2003;162:55-56.

[78]   Proujansky, R; Winter, HS; Walker, WA. Gastrointestinal syndromes associated with food sensitivity. *Adv. Pediatr.* 1988;35:219-238.

[79]   Troncone, R; Discepolo, V. Colon in food allergy. *J Pediatr Gastroentrol Nutr.* 2009;48 (Suppl 2):S89-91.

[80]   Troncone, R; Bhatnagar, S; Butzner, D; et al. Celiac disease and other immunologically mediated disorders of the gastrointestinal tract: Working Group Report of the Second World Congress of Pediatric Gastroenterology, Hepatology, and Nutrition. *J. Pediatr. Gastroenterol. Nutr.* 2004;39:S601-S610.

[81]   Dewar, DH; Ciclitira, PJ. Clinical features and diagnosis of celiac disease. *Gastroenterology.* 2005;128:S19-S24.

[82]   Estep, DC; Kulczycki, A, Jr. Treatment of infant colic with amino acid-based infant formula: a preliminary study. *Acta Paediatr.* 2000;89:22-27.

[83]   Hill, DJ; Hudson, IL; Sheffield, LJ; et al. A low allergen diet is a significant intervention in infantile colic: results of a community-based study. *J. Allergy Clin. Immunol.* 1995;96:886-892.

[84]   Iacono, G; Carroccio, A; Montalto, G; et al. Severe infantile colic and food intolerance: a long-term prospective study. *J. Pediatr. Gastroenterol. Nutr.* 1991;12:332-335.

[85]   Leung, AK; Lemay, JF. Infantile colic: a review. *J. R. Soc. Health.* 2004;124:162-166.

[86]   Lothe, L; Lindberg, T. Cow's milk whey protein elicits symptoms of infantile colic in colicky formula-fed infants: a double-blind crossover study. *Pediatrics*. 1989;83:262-266.

[87]   Lucassen, PL; Assendelft, WJ; Gubbels, JW; et al. Infantile colic: crying time reduction with a whey hydrolysate: a double-blind, randomized, placebo-controlled trial. *Pediatrics*. 2000;106:1349-1354.

[88]   Savino, F. Focus on infantile colic. *Acta Paediatr*. 2007;96:1259-1264.

[89]   Hill, DJ; Hosking, CS. Infantile colic and food hypersensitivity. *J. Pediatr. Gastroenterol. Nutr*. 2000;30:S67-S76.

[90]   Kalliomäki, M; Lappala, P; Korvenranta, H; et al. Extent of fussing and colic type crying preceding atopic disease. *Arch. Dis. Child*. 2001;84:349-350.

[91]   Jakobsson, I; Lothe, L; Ley, D; et al. Effectiveness of casein hydrolysate feedings in infants with colic. *Acta Paediatr*. 2000; 89:18-21.

[92]   Jakobbson, I; Lindberg, T. Cow's milk proteins cause infantile colic in breast-fed infants: a double-blind crossover study. *Pediatrics*. 1983;71:268-271.

[93]   Hewson, P; Oberklaid, F; Menahem, S. Infant colic, distress, and crying. *Clin. Pediatr*. 1987;26:69-75.

[94]   Nutrition Committee, Canadian Paediatric Society. Dietary manipulations for infantile colic. *Paediatr. Child Health*. 2003;8:449-452.

[95]   Hill, DJ; Roy, N; Heine, RG; et al. Effect of a low-allergen maternal diet on colic among breastfed infants: a randomized, controlled trial. *Pediatrics*. 2005;116:e709-e715.

[96]   Kalliomäki, MA. Food allergy and irritable bowel syndrome. *Curr. Opin. Gastroenterol*. 2005;21:708-711.

[97]   Park, MI; Camilleri, M. Is there a role of food allergy in irritable bowel syndrome and functional dyspepsia? A systemic review. *Neurogastroenterol. Motil*. 2006;18:595-607.

[98]   Gonsalkorale, WM; Perrey, C; Pravica, V; et al. Interleukin 10 genotypes in irritable bowel syndrome: evidence for an inflammatory component? *Gut*. 2003;52:91-93.

[99]   van der Veek, PP; van den Berg, M; de Kroon, YE; et al. Role of tumor necrosis factor-α and interleukin-10 gene polymorphisms in irritable bowel syndrome. *Am. J. Gastroenterol*. 2005;100:2510-2516.

[100] Barbara, G; Stanghellini, V; de Giorgio, R; et al. Activated mast cells in proximity to colonic nerves correlate with abdominal pain in irritable bowel syndrome. *Gastroenterology.* 2004;126:693-702.

[101] Atkinson, W; Sheldon, TA; Shaath, N; et al. Food elimination based on IgG antibodies in irritable bowel syndrome: a randomized controlled trial. *Gut.* 2004;53:1459-1464.

[102] Isolauri, E; Rautava, S; Kalliomäki, M. Food allergy in irritable bowel syndrome: new facts and old fallacies. *Gut.* 2004;53:1391-1393.

[103] Leung, AK; Wong, BE; Cho, HY, et al. Recurrent abdominal pain in childhood. *Singapore Pediatr. J.* 1996;38:44-48.

[104] Leung, AK; Lemay, JF; Barker, C. Recurrent abdominal pain in children. *Can. J. Diagn.* 2002;19(5):68-80.

[105] Kokkonen, J; Ruuska, T; Karttunen, T; et al. Mucosal pathology of the foregut associating with food allergy and recurrent abdominal pains in children. *Acta Paediatr.* 2001;90:16-21.

[106] Husby, S; Host, A. Recurrent abdominal pain, food allergy and endoscopy. *Acta Paediatr.* 2001;90:3-4.

[107] Leung, AK; Chan, PY; Cho, HY. Constipation in children. *Am. Fam. Physician.* 1996;54:611-627.

[108] Loening-Baucke, V. Prevalence, symptoms and outcome of constipation in infants and toddlers. *J. Pediatr.* 2005;146:359-363.

[109] Iacono, G; Carroccio, A; Cavataio, F; et al. Chronic constipation as a symptom of cow milk allergy. *J. Pediatr.* 1995;126:34-39.

[110] Iacono, G; Cavataio, F; Montalto,G; et al. Intolerance of cow's milk and chronic constipation in children. *N. Engl. J. Med.* 1998;339:1100-1104.

[111] Daher, S; Tahan, S; Solé, D; et al. Cow's milk protein intolerance and chronic constipation in children. *Pediatr. Allergy Immunol.* 2001;1:339-342.

[112] Carroccio, A; Scalici, C; Maresi, E; et al. Chronic constipation and food intolerance: a model of proctitis causing constipation. *Scand. J. Gastroenterol.* 2005;40:33-42.

[113] Burks, W. Skin manifestations of food allergy. *Pediatrics.* 2003;111:1617-1624.

[114] Fasano, MB. Dermatologic food allergy. *Pediatr. Ann.* 2006;35:727-731.

[115] Host, A; Halken, S. A prospective study of cow milk allergy in Danish infants during the first 3 years of life. *Allergy.* 1990;45:587-596.

[116] Hill, DJ; Firer, MA; Shelton, MJ; et al. Manifestations of milk allergy in infants: clinical and immunologic findings. *J. Pediatr.* 1986;109:270-276.

[117] Champion, RH; Roberts, SO; Carpenter RG; et al: Urticaria and angioedema: a review of 554 patients. *Br. J. Dermatol.* 1969;81:588-597.

[118] Lemanske, RF Jr.; Sampson, HA. Adverse reactions to foods and their relationships to skin diseases in children. *Adv. Pediatr.* 1988;35: 89-218.

[119] Winston, GB; Lewis, CW. Contact dermatitis. *Int. J. Dermatol.* 1982;21:573-578.

[120] Pastar, Z; Lipozencic, J. Adverse reactions to food and clinical expressions of food allergy. *SKINmed.* 2006;5:119-125.

[121] Sampson, HA. The immunopathogenic role of food hypersensitivity in atopic dermatitis. *Acta Derm. Venereol.* 1992;176:S34-S37.

[122] Gontzes, P; Bahna, SL. Food allergy for the primary care physician. *Primary Care.* 1987;14:547-558.

[123] Leung, AK; Hon, KL; Robson, WL. Atopic dermatitis. *Adv. Pediatr.* 2007;54:241-273.

[124] Burks, AW; Mallroy, SB; Williams, LW; et al. Atopic dermatitis: clinical relevance of food hypersensitivity reactions. *J. Pediatr.* 1988;113:447-451.

[125] Sampson, HA; McCaskill, CC. Food hypersensitivity and atopic dermatitis: evaluation of 113 patients. *J. Pediatr.* 1985;107:669-675.

[126] Sampson, HA; Mendelson, L; Rosen, JP. Fatal and near-fatal anaphylactic reactions to food in children and adolescents. *N. Engl. J. Med.* 1992;327:380-384.

[127] Breuer, K; Heratizadeh, A; Wulf, A; et al. Late eczematous reactions to food in children with atopic dermatitis. *Clin. Exp. Allergy.* 2004;34:817-824.

[128] Hill, DJ; Hosking, CS. Food allergy and atopic dermatitis in infancy: an epidemiology study. *Pediatr. Allergy Immunol.* 2004;15:421-427.

[129] Dolovich, J; Hargreave, FE; Chalmers, R; et al. Late cutaneous allergic responses in isolated IgE-dependent reactions. *J. Allergy Clin. Immunol.* 1973;52:38-46.

[130] Solley, GO; Gleich, GJ; Jordan, RE; et al. The late phase of the immediate wheal and flare skin reactions: its dependence on IgE antibodies. *J. Clin. Invest.* 1976;58:408-420.

[131] Lio, PA. Atopic dermatitis and food allergies: true, true and related? *Arch. Dis. Child. Educ. Pract. Ed.* 2007;92:ep56-ep60.

[132] Hill, DJ; Duke, AM; Hosking, CS; et al. Clinical manifestations of cow's milk allergy in childhood. II. The diagnostic value of skin tests and RAST. *Clin. Allergy.* 1988;18:481-490.

[133] Brancaccio, RR; Alvarez, MS. Contact allergy to food. *Dermatol. Ther.* 2004;17:302-313.

[134] Judd, L. A descriptive study of occupational skin disease. *N. Z. Med. J.* 1994;107:147-149.

[135] Ekeowa-Anderson, AL. Allergic contact cheilitis to garlic. *Contact Dermatitis.* 2007;56:174-175.

[136] Tamagawa-Mineoka, R; Katoh, N; Kishimoto, S. Allergic contact cheilitis due to geraniol in food. *Contact Dermatitis.* 2007;56:242-243.

[137] Hall, RP. Dermatitis herpetiformis. *J. Invest. Dermatol.* 1992;99:873-881.

[138] Solheim, BG; Ek, J; Thune, PO; et al. HLA antigens in dermatitis herpetiformis and coeliac disease. *Tissue Antigens.* 1976;7:57-59.

[139] El-Gamal, YM; Hossny, EM. Respiratory food allergy. *Pediatr. Ann.* 2006;35:733-740.

[140] James, JM. Respiratory manifestations of food allergy. *Pediatrics.* 2003;111:1625-1630.

[141] Burks, AW; Sampson, H. Food allergies in children. *Curr. Probl. Pediatr.* 1993;23:230-252.

[142] Ortolani, C. Atlas on mechanisms in adverse reactions to food. *Allergy.* 1995;50:5-81.

[143] James, JM; Crespo, JF. Allergic reactions to foods by inhalation. *Curr. Allergy Asthma Rep.* 2007;7:167-174.

[144] Ozol, D; Mete, E. Asthma and food allergy. *Curr. Opin. Pulm. Med.* 2008;14:9-12.

[145] Onorato, J; Merland, N; Terral, C; et al: Placebo-controlled double-blind food challenge in asthma. *J. Allergy Clin. Immunol.* 1986;78:1139-1146.

[146] Roberts, G; Lack, G. Food allergy and asthma – what is the link? *Paediatr. Respir. Rev.* 2003;4:205-212.

[147] Rance, F; Micheau, P; Marchac, V; et al. Food allergy and asthma in children. *Rev. Pneumol. Clin.* 2003;59:109-113

[148] James, JM; Eggleston, PA; Sampson, HA. Food allergy increases airway reactivity. *Am. J. Crit. Care Respir. Med.* 1994;149:59-64.

[149] Roberts, G; Lack, G. Relevance of inhalational exposure to food allergens. *Curr. Opin. Allergy Clin. Immunol.* 2003;3:211-215.

[150] Crespo, JF; Pascual, C; Dominguez, C; et al. Allergic reactions associated with airborne fish particles in IgE-mediated fish hypersensitive patients. *Allergy.* 1995;50:257-261.

[151] Roberts, G; Golder, N; Lack, G. Bronchial challenges with aerosolized food in asthmatic, food-allergic children. *Allergy.* 2002;57:713-717.

[152] Sicherer, SH; Furlong, TJ; DeSimone, J; et al. Self-reported allergic reactions to peanuts on commercial airlines. *J. Allergy Clin. Immunol.* 1999;104:186-189.

[153] Gustafsson, D; Sjöberg, O; Foucard, T. Sensitization to food and airborne allergens in children with atopic dermatitis followed up to 7 years of age. *Pediatr. Allergy Immunol.* 2003;14:448-452.

[154] Kotaniemi-Syrjanen, A; Reijonen, T; Romppanen, J. Allergen-specific immunoglobulin E antibodies in wheezing infants: the risk for asthma in later childhood. *Pediatrics.* 2003;111:e255-e261.

[155] Simpson, AB; Glutting, J; Yousef, E. Food allergy and asthma morbidity in children. *Pediatr. Pulmonol.* 2007;42:489-495.

[156] Heiner, DC; Sears, JW. Chronic respiratory disease associated with multiple circulating precipitins to cow's milk. *Am. J. Dis. Child.* 1960;100:500-502.

[157] Bahna, SL. Adverse food reactions by skin contact. *Allergy.* 2004;59(Suppl 78):66-70.

[158] Aydoğan, B; Kiroğlu, M; Altintas, D; et al. The role of food allergy in otitis media with effusion. *Otolaryngol. Head Neck Surg.* 2004;130:747-750.

[159] Bernstein, JM; Lee, J; Conboy, K; et al. Further observations on the role of IgE-mediated hypersensitivity in recurrent otitis media with effusion. *Otolaryngol. Head Neck Surg.* 1985;93:611-615.

[160] Luyasu, S; Morisset, M; Guenard, L; et al. Acute recurrent otalgia and food allergy: a case report and review of the literature. *Eur. Ann. Allergy Clin. Immunol.* 2005;37:60-62.

[161] Nsouli, TM; Nsouli, SM; Linde, RE; et al. Role of food allergy in serous otitis media. *Ann. Allergy.* 1994;73:215-219.

[162] Juntti, H; Tikkanen, S; Kokkonen, J; et al. Cow's milk allergy is associated with recurrent otitis media during childhood. *Acta Otolaryngol.* 1999;119:867-873.

[163] Derebery, MJ; Berliner, KI. Prevalence of allergy in Meniere's disease. *Otolaryngol. Head Neck Surg.* 2000;123:69-75.

[164] Keleş, E; Gödekmerdan, A; Kalidağ, T; et al. Ménière's disease and allergy: allergens and cytokines. *J. Laryngol. Otol.* 2004;118:688-693.

[165] Monro, J; Carini, C; Brostoff, J. Migraine is a food-allergic disease. *Lancet.* 1984;1:719-721.

[166] Mansfield, LE; Vaughan, TR; Waller, SF; et al. Food allergy and adult migraine: double-blind and mediator confirmation of an allergic etiology. *Ann. Allergy.* 1985;55:126-129.

[167] Egger, J; Carter, CM; Soothill, JF; et al. Oligoantigenic diet treatment of children with epilepsy and migraine. *J. Pediatr.* 1989;114:51-58.

[168] Stern, M. Allergic enteropathy. In: Walker, WA; Durie, PR; Hamilton, JR; et al. (eds). *Pediatric Gastrointestinal Disease.* St Louis: Mosby. 1996; pp. 677-692.

[169] Fotherby, KJ; Hunter, JO. Symptoms of food allergy. *Clin. Gastroenterol.* 1985;14:615-629.

[170] Pearson, DJ; McKee, A. Food allergy. *Adv. Nutr. Res.* 1985;7:1-37.

[171] Johansson, SG; Hourihane, JO; Bousquet, J; et al. A revised nomenclature for allergy. An EAACI position statement from the EAACI nomenclature task force. *Allergy.* 2001;56:813-824.

[172] Crayton, JW; Stone, T; Stein, G. Epilepsy precipitated by food sensitivity: report of a case with double-blind placebo-controlled assessment. *Clin. Electroencephalographol.* 1981;12:192-198.

[173] Frediani, T; Lucarelli, S; Pelliccia, A; et al. Allergy and childhood epilepsy: a close relationship? *Acta Neurol. Scand.* 2001;104:349-352.

[174] Frediani, T; Pelliccia, A; Aprile, A; et al. Partial idiopathic epilepsy: recovery after allergen-free diet. *Pediatr. Med. Chir.* 2004;26:196-197.

[175] Cavallo, MG; Fava, D; Monetini, L; et al. Cell-mediated immune response to ß casein in recent-onset insulin-dependent diabetes: implications for disease pathogenesis. *Lancet.* 1996;348:926-928.

[176] Harrison, LC. Cow's milk and IDDM. *Lancet.* 1996;348:905-906.

[177] Karjalainen, J; Martin, JM; Knip, M; et al. A bovine albumin peptide as a possible trigger of insulin-dependent diabetes mellitus. *N. Engl. J. Med.* 1992;327:302-307.

[178] Norris, JM; Beaty, B; Klingensmith, G; et al. Lack of association between early exposure to cow's milk protein and ß-cell autoimmunity: diabetes autoimmunity study in the young (DAISY). *JAMA.* 1996;276:609-614.

[179] Sandberg, DH; McIntosh, RM; Bernstein, CW; et al. Severe steroid-responsive nephrosis associated with hypersensitivity. *Lancet.* 1997;1:388-391.

[180] Genova, R; Sanfilippo, M; Rossi, ME; et al. Food allergy in steroid-resistant nephrotic syndrome. *Lancet.* 1987;1:1315-1316.

[181] Laurent, J; Rostoker, G; Robera, R; et al. Is adult idiopathic nephrotic syndrome food allergy? Value of oligoantigenic diets. *Nephron.* 1987;47:7-11.

[182] Sieniawska, M; Szymanik-Grzelak, H; Kowalewska, M; et al. The role of cow's milk protein intolerance in steroid-resistant nephrotic syndrome. *Acta Paediatr.* 1992;81:1007-1012.

[183] Whitefield, MF; Barr, DGD. Cow's milk allergy in the syndrome of thrombocytopenia with absent radius. *Arch. Dis. Child.* 1976;51:337-343.

[184] Jones, RHT. Congenital thrombocytopenia and milk allergy. *Arch. Dis. Child.* 1977;52:744-745.

[185] Caffrey, EA; Sladen, GE; Isaacs, PET; et al: Thrombocytopenia caused by cow's milk. *Lancet.* 1981;2:316.

[186] Businco, L; Falconieri, P; Bellioni-Businco, B; et al. Severe food-induced vasculitis in two children. *Pediatr. Allergy Immunol.* 2002;12:68-71.

[187] Lunardi, C; Bambara, LM; Biasi, D; et al. Elimination diet in the treatment of selected patients with hypersensitivity vasculitis. *Clin. Exp .Rheum.* 1992;10:131-135.

[188] Panush, RS; Carter, RL; Katz, P; et al. Diet therapy for rheumatoid arthritis. *Arthritis Rheum.* 1983;26:462-471.

[189] Panush, RS; Stroud, RM; Webster, EM. Food-induced (allergic) arthritis: Inflammatory arthritis exacerbated by milk. *Arthritis Rheum.* 1986;29:220-226.

[190] Panush, RS. Food induced ("allergic") arthritis: clinical and serologic studies. *J. Rheumatol.* 1990;17:291-294.

[191] Parke, AL; Hughes, GR. Rheumatoid arthritis and food: a case study. *Br. Med. J.* 1981;282:2027-2029.

[192] Golding, DN. Is there an allergic synovitis? *J. R. Soc. Med.* 1990;83:312-314.

[193] van der Laar, MA; van der Korst, JK. Food intolerance in rheumatoid arthritis. I. A double blind, controlled trial of the clinical effects of elimination of milk allergens and azo dyes. *Ann. Rheum. Dis.* 1992;51:298-302.

[194] Denman, AM; Mitchell, B; Ansell, BM. Joint complaints and food allergic disorders. *Ann. Allergy.* 1983;51:260-263.

[195] Karatay, S; Erdem, T; Yildirim, K; et al. The effect of individualized diet challenges consisting of allergenic foods on TNF-α and IL-1β levels in patients with rheumatoid arthritis. *Rheumatology.* 2004;43:1429-1433.

[196] Bock, SA; Buckley, J; Holst, A; et al. Proper use of skin tests with food extracts in diagnosis of hypersensitivity to food in children. *Clin. Allergy.* 1977;7:375 -383.

[197] Sampson, HA. Food allergy. Part 2: diagnosis and management. *J. Allergy Clin. Immunol.* 1999;103:981-99.

[198] Sampson HA. Utility of food-specific IgE concentrations in predicting symptomatic food allergy. *J. Allergy Clin. Immunol.* 2001;107: 891-896.

[199] Bock, SA. Prospective appraisal of complaints of adverse reactions to foods in children during the first 3 years of life. *Pediatrics.* 1987;79:683-688.

[200] Burks, AW; Ballmer-Weber, BK. Food allergies. *Mol. Nutr. Food Res.* 2006;50:595-603.

[201] Nieuwenhuizen, N; Lopata, A. Fighting food allergy: current approaches. *Ann. N. Y. Acad. Sci.* 2005;1056:30-45.

[202] Lee, LA; Burks, AW. Food allergies: prevalence, molecular characterization, and treatment/prevention strategies. *Annu. Rev. Nutr.* 2006;26;539-565.

[203] Bock, SA; Munoz-Furlong, A; Sampson, HA. Fatalities due to anaphylactic reactions to foods. *J. Allergy Clin. Immunol.* 2001;107:191-193.

[204] Fiocchi, A; Martelli, A. Dietary management of food allergy. *Pediatr. Ann.* 2006;35:755-763.

[205] James, JM; Crespo, JF. Allergic reactions to foods by inhalation. *Curr. Allergy Asthma Rep.* 2007;7:167-174.

[206] Nowak-Wegrzyn, A. Immunotherapy for food allergy. *Inflamm. Allergy Drug Targets.* 2006;5:23-34.

[207] Altman, DR; Chiaramonte, LT. Public perception of food allergy. *J. Allergy Clin. Immunol.* 1996;97:1247-1251.

[208] Opper, PH; Burakoff, R. Food allergy and intolerance. *Gastroenterologist.* 1993;1:211-220.

[209] Sicherer, SH; Leung, DY. Advances in allergic skin disease, anaphylaxis, and hypersensitivity reactions to foods, drugs, and insects. *J. Allergy Clin. Immunol.* 2007;119:1462-1469.

[210] Venter, C; Pereira, B; Grundy, J; et al. Incidence of parentally reported and clinically diagnosed food hypersensitivity in the first year of life. *J. Allergy Clin. Immunol.* 2006;117:1118-1124.

[211] Grimshaw, KE. Dietary management of food allergy in children. *Proc. Nutr. Soc.* 2006;65:412-417.

[212] Joint Task Force on Practice Parameters; American Academy of Allergy, Asthma and Immunology; American College of Allergy, Asthma and Immunology; Joint Council of Allergy, Asthma and Immunology. The diagnosis and management of anaphylaxis: an updated practice parameter. *J. Allergy Clin. Immunol.* 2005;115:S483-S523.

[213] Muñoz-Furlong, A. Daily coping strategies for patients and their families. *Pediatrics.* 2003;111:1654-1661.

[214] Joshi, P; Mofidi, S; Sicherer, SH. Interpretation of commercial food ingredient labels by parents of food-allergic children. *J. Allergy Clin. Immunol.* 2002;109:1019-1021.

[215] Taylor, SL; Hefle, SL. Food allergen labeling in the USA and Europe. *Curr. Opin. Allergy Clin. Immunol.* 2006;6:186-190.

[216] European Commission. Directive 2003/89/EC of the European Parliament and of the Council of 10 November 2003 amending Directive 2000/13/EC as regards indication of the ingredients present in foodstuffs. *Official J. Euro. Communities.* 2003;308:15-18.

[217] Lee, BW. Food and allergy. *Ann. Acad. Med. Singapore.* 1995;24:238-241.

[218] Steinman, HA. "Hidden" allergens in foods. *J. Allergy Clin. Immunol.* 1996;98:241-250.

[219] Dannaeus, A. Food allergy in infancy and children. *Ann. Allergy.* 1987;59:124-126.

[220] Leung, AK; Bowen, TJ. Seasonal allergic rhinitis and food allergy. In: Bergman, AB. (ed). *Twenty Common Problems in Pediatrics.* New York: McGraw-Hill. 2001, pp. 219-233.

[221] Oren, E; Banerji, A; Clark, S; et al. Food-induced anaphylaxis and repeated epinephrine treatments. *Ann. Allergy Asthma Immunol.* 2007;99:429-432.

[222] Kelso, JM. A second dose of epinephrine for anaphylaxis: how often needed and how to carry. *J. Allergy Clin. Immunol.* 2006;117:464-465.

[223] Clark, S; Camargo, CA, Jr. Emergency management of food allergy: systems perspective. *Curr. Opin. Allergy Clin. Immunol.* 2005;5:293-298.

[224] Baral, VR; Hourihane, JO. Food allergy in children. *Postgrad. Med. J.* 2005;81:693-701.

[225] Muraro, A; Roberts, G; Clark, A; et al. The management of anaphylaxis in childhood: position paper of the European Academy of Allergology and Clinical Immunology. *Allergy.* 2007;62:857-871.

[226] Wang, J; Sampson, HA. Food anaphylaxis. *Clin. Exp. Allergy.* 2007;37:651-660.

[227] Simons, FE; Roberts, JR; Gu, X; et al. Epinephrine absorption in children with a history of anaphylaxis. *J. Allergy Clin. Immunol.* 1998;101:33-37.

[228] Brown, SG. Cardiovascular aspects of anaphylaxis: implications for treatment and diagnosis. *Curr. Opin. Allergy Clin. Immunol.* 2005;5:359-364.

[229] Simons, FE. First-aid treatment of anaphylaxis to food: focus on epinephrine. *J. Allergy Clin. Immunol.* 2004;113:837-844.

[230] Du Toit, G; Fox, A; Morris, A. Managing food allergy in children. *Practitioner.* 2006;250:45-46, 49-52.

[231] Metcalfe, DD. Food hypersensitivity. *J. Allergy Clin. Immunol.* 1984;73:749-762.

[232] Leung, AK; Hon, KL; Robson, WL. Atopic dermatitis. *Adv. Pediatr.* 2007;54:241-273.

[233] Bailey, M; Haverson, K; Inman, C; et al. The development of the mucosal immune system pre- and post-weaning: balancing regulatory and effector function. *Proc. Nutr. Soc.* 2005;64:451-457.

[234] Kalliomäki, M; Kirjavainen, P; Eerola, E; et al. Distinct patterns of neonatal gut microflora in infants in whom atopy was and was not developing. *J. Allergy Clin. Immunol.* 2001;107:129-134.

[235] Watanabe, S; Narisawa, Y; Arase, S; et al. Differences in fecal microflora between patients with atopic dermatitis and healthy control subjects. *J. Allergy Clin. Immunol.* 2003;111:587-591.

[236] Björkstén, B; Sepp, E; Julge,K; et al. Allergy development and the intestinal microflora during the first year of life. *J. Allergy Clin. Immunol.* 2001;108:516-520.

[237] Laitenen, K; Isolauri, E. Management of food allergy: vitamins, fatty acids or probiotics? *Eur. J. Gastroenterol. Hepatol.* 2005;17:1305-1311.

[238] Boyle, RJ; Tang, ML. The role of probiotics in the management of allergic disease. *Clin. Exp. Allergy.* 2006;36:568-576.

[239] He, F; Morita, H; Hashimoto, H; et al. Intestinal *Bifidobacterium* species induce varying cytokine production. *J. Allergy Clin. Immunol.* 2002;109:1035-1036.

[240] Kirjavainen, PV; Apostolou, E; Salminen, SJ, et al. New aspects of probiotics – a novel approach in the management of food allergy. *Allergy.* 1999;54:909-915.

[241] O'Sullivan, GC; Kelly, P; O'Halloran, S; et al. Probiotics: an emerging therapy. *Curr. Pharm. Des.* 2005;11:3-10.

[242] Rosenfeld, V; Benfeldt, E; Valerius, NH; et al. Effect of probiotics on gastrointestinal symptoms and small intestinal permeability in children with atopic dermatitis. *J. Pediatr.* 2004;145:612-616

[243] Williams, HC. Two "positive" studies of probiotics for atopic dermatitis – or are they? *Arch. Dermatol.* 2006;142:1201-1203.

[244] Kalliomäki, M; Salminen, S; Arvilommi, H; et al. Probiotics in primary prevention of atopic disease: a randomized placebo-controlled trial. *Lancet.* 2001;357:1076-1079.

[245] Kalliomäki, M; Salminen, S; Poussa, T; et al. Probiotics and prevention of atopic disease: 4-year follow-up of a randomized placebo-controlled trial. *Lancet.* 2003;361:1869-1871.

[246] Lodinová-Zádníková, R; Cukrowska, B; Tlaskalova-Hogenova, H. Oral administration of probiotic *Escherichia coli* after birth reduces frequency of allergies and repeated infections later in life (after 10 and 20 years). *Int. Arch. Allergy Immunol.* 2003;131:209-211.

[247] Rosenfeld, V; Benfeldt, E; Nielsen, SD; et al. Effect of probiotic *lactobacilli* strains in children with atopic dermatitis. *J. Allergy Clin. Immunol.* 2003;111:389-395.

[248] Viljanen, M; Savilahti, E; Haahtela, T; et al. Probiotics in the treatment of atopic eczema/dermatitis syndrome in infants: a double-blind placebo-controlled trial. *Allergy.* 2005;60:494-500.

[249] Tamura, M; Shikina, T; Morihana, T; et al. Effects of probiotics on allergic rhinitis induced by Japanese cedar pollen: randomized double-blind, placebo-controlled clinical trial. *Int. Arch. Allergy Immunol.* 2007;143:75-82.

[250] Taylor, AL; Dunstan, JA; Prescott, SL, et al. Probiotic supplementation for the first 6 months of life fails to reduce the risk of atopic dermatitis and increases the risk of allergen sensitization in high-risk children: a randomized controlled trial. *J. Allergy Clin. Immunol.* 2007;119:184-191.

[251] Kukkonen, K; Savilahti, E; Haahtela, T; et al. Probiotic and prebiotic galacto-oligosaccharides in the prevention of allergic diseases: a randomized, double-blind, placebo-controlled trial. *J. Allergy Clin. Immunol.* 2007;119:192-198.

[252] Weston, S; Halbert, A; Richmond, P; et al. Effects of probiotics on atopic dermatitis: a randomized controlled trial. *Arch. Dis. Child.* 2005;90:892-897.

[253] Passeron, T; Lacour, JP; Fontas, E; et al. Prebiotics and synbiotics: two promising approaches for the treatment of atopic dermatitis in children above 2 years. *Allergy.* 2006;61:431-437.

[254] Greer, FR; Sicherer, SH; Burks, AW; and the Committee on Nutrition and Section on Allergy and Immunology. Effects of early nutritional interventions on the development of atopic disease in infants and children: The role of maternal dietary restriction, breastfeeding, timing of introduction of complementary foods and hydrolyzed formulas. *Pediatrics.* 2008;121:183-191.

[255] Greer, FR; Sicherer, SH; Burks, AW. Effects of early nutritional interventions on the development of atopic disease in infants and children: the role of maternal dietary restriction, breastfeeding, timing of introduction of complementary foods, and hydrolyzed formulas. *Pediatrics.* 2008; 121:183-91.

[256] Zeiger, RS; Heller, S. The development and prediction of atopy in high-risk children: follow-up at age seven years in a prospective randomized study of combined maternal and infant food allergen avoidance. *J. Allergy Clin. Immunol.* 1995; 95:1179-90.

[257] Björkstén, B; Kjellman, NI. Does breast-feeding prevent food allergy? *Allergy Proc.* 1991;12:233-237.

[258] Bahna, SL. Management of food allergies. *Ann. Allergy.* 1984;53:678-682.

[259] Kramer, MS; Kakuma, R. Maternal dietary antigen avoidance during pregnancy and/or lactation for preventing or treating atopic disease in the child. *Cochrane Database Syst. Rev.* 2006;(3): CD000133

[260] Zutavern, A; Brockow, I; Schaaf, B; et al. Timing of solid food introduction in relation to eczema, asthma, allergic rhinitis, and food and inhalant sensitization at the age of 6 years: results from the prospective birth cohort study LISA. *Pediatrics.* 2008;121:e44-e52.

[261] Kull, I; Bergestro, A; Lilja, G; et al. Fish consumption during the first year of life and development of allergic diseases during childhood. *Allergy.* 2006;61:1009-1015.

[262] Poole, JA; Barriga, K; Donald, Y; et al. Timing of initial exposure to cereal grains and the risk of wheat allergy. *Pediatrics.* 2006;117:2175-2182.

[263] Fiocchi, A; Assa'ad, A; Bahna, S; et al. Food allergy and the introduction of solid foods to infants: a consensus document. Adverse Reactions to Foods Committee, American College of Allergy, Asthma and Immunology. *Ann Allergy Asthma Immunol.* 2006;97(1):10-20

[264] Hodge, L; Salome, CM; Peat, JK; et al. Consumption of oily fish and childhood asthma risk. *Med. J. Aust.* 1998;164:137-140.

[265] Mayser, P; Mayer, K; Mahloudjian, M; et al. A double-blind, randomized, placebo-controlled trial of n-3 versus n-6 fatty acid-based lipid infusion in atopic dermatitis. *J. Parent. Enter. Nutr.* 2002;26:151-158.

[266] Nafstad, P; Nystad, W; Magnus, P; et al. Asthma and allergic rhinitis at 4 years of age in relation to fish consumption in infancy. *J. Asthma.* 2003;40:343-348.

[267] Thien, FCK; Woods, R; de Lucas S; et al. Dietary marine fatty acids (fish oil) for asthma in adults and children. *Cochrane Database Sys. Rev.* 2002;3:CD001283.

[268] Gool, CJ; Zeegers, MP; Thijs, C. Oral essential fatty acid supplementation in atopic dermatitis – a meta-analysis of placebo-controlled trials. *Br. J. Dermatol.* 2004;150:728-740.

[269] Host, A; Halken, S. Primary prevention of food allergy in infants who are at risk. *Curr. Opin. Allergy Clin. Immunol.* 2005;5:255-259.

[270] Hays, T; Wood, RA. A systematic review of the role of hydrolysed infant formulas in allergy prevention. *Arch. Pediatr. Adolesc. Med.* 2005;159:810-816.

[271] Osborn, DA; Sinn, J. Formulas containing hydrolysed protein for prevention of allergy and food intolerance in infants (review). *Cochrane Database Syst. Rev.* 2006 18;(4):CD003664.

[272] Zeiger, RS. Food allergen avoidance in the prevention of food allergy in infancy and children. *Pediatrics.* 2003;111:1662-1671.

[273] Osborn, DA; Sinn, J. Soy formula for prevention of allergy and food intolerance in infants (review). *Cochrane Database Syst. Rev.* 2006;4:CD003741.

[274] American Academy of Pediatrics, Committee on Nutrition. Hypoallergenic infant formulas. *Pediatrics.* 2000;106:346-349.

[275] Siltanen, M; Kajosaari, M; Poussa, T; et al. A dual long-term effect of breastfeeding on atopy in relation to heredity in children at 4 years of age. *Allergy.* 2003;58:524-530.

[276] Kajosaari, M; Saarinen, UM. Prophylaxis of atopic disease by six months' total solid foods elimination. *Acta Paediatr. Scand.* 1983;72:411-421.

[277] Morgan, J; Williams, P; Norris, F; et al. Eczema and early solid feeding in preterm infants. *Arch. Dis. Child.* 2004;89:309-314.

[278] Fiocchi, A; Assa'ad, A; Bahna, S; et al. Food allergy and the introduction of solid foods to infants: a consensus document. *Ann. Allergy Asthma Immunol.* 2006;97:10-21.

[279] Marini, A; Agosti, M; Motta, G; et al. Effects of a dietary and environmental prevention programme on the incidence of allergic symptoms in high atopic risk infants: three years follow-up. *Acta Paediatr.* 1996;414:S1-S22.

[280] Halken, S; Host, A; Hansen, LG; et al. Effect of an allergy prevention programme on incidence of atopic symptoms in infancy: a prospective study of 159 "high-risk" infants. *Allergy.* 1992;47:545-553.

[281] Leung, AK; Sauve, RS. Whole cow's milk in infancy. *Paediatr. Child. Health.* 2003;8:419-421.

[282] Duggan, C; Walker, WA. Protein intolerance. In: Oski, FA; DeAngelis, CD; Feigin, RD. (eds). *Principles and Practice of Pediatrics.* Philadelphia: JB Lippincott. 1994; pp.1887-1890.

[283] Rozenfeld, P; Docena GH; Anon, MC; et al. Detection and identification of a soy protein that cross-reacts with caseins from cow's milk. *Clin Exp Immunol.* 2002;130:49-58.

[284] Crittenden, RG; Bennett, LE. Cow's milk allergy: a complex disorder. *J. Am. Coll. Nutr.* 2005;24:S582-S591.

[285] Bellioni-Businco, B; Paganelli, R; Lucenti, P; et al. Allergenicity of goat's milk in children with cow's milk allergy. *J. Allergy Clin. Immunol.* 1999;103:1191-1194.

[286] Committee on Nutrition, American Academy of Pediatrics. Food sensitivity. In: Kleinman, RE. (ed). *Pediatric Nutrition Handbook.* Elk Grove Village, Ill: American Academy of Pediatrics. 2004; pp.593-607.

[287] Sampson, HA; Bernhisel-Broadbent, J; Yang, E; et al. Safety of casein hydrolysate formula in children with cow milk allergy. *J. Pediatr.* 1991;118:520-525

[288] Sampson, HA; James, JM; Bernhisel-Broadbent, J. Safety of an amino acid-derived infant formula in children allergic to cow's milk. *Pediatrics.* 1992;90:463-465.

[289] Chehade, M; Magid, MS; Mofidi, S; et al. Allergic eosinophilic gastroenteritis with protein-losing enteropathy: intestinal pathology, clinical course, and long-term follow-up. *J. Pediatr. Gastroenterol. Nutr.* 2006;42:516-521.

[290] Kagalwalla, AF; Sentongo, TA; Ritz, S; et al. Effect of six-food elimination diet on clinical and histologic outcomes in eosinophilic esophagitis. *Clin. Gastroenterol. Hepatol.* 2006;4:1097-1102.

[291] Liacouras, CA. Eosinophilic esophagitis: treatment in 2005. *Curr. Opin. Gastroenterol.* 2006;22:147-142.

[292] Nelson, HS; Lahr, J; Rule, R, et al. Treatment of anaphylactic sensitivity to peanuts by immunotherapy with injections of aqueous peanuts extract. *J. Allergy Clin. Immunol.* 1997;99:744-751.

[293] Pons, L; Burks, W. Novel treatments for food allergy. *Expert Opin. Investig. Drugs.* 2005;14:829-834.

[294] Allen, KJ; Hill, DJ, Heine, RG. 4. Food allergy in childhood. *MJA.* 2006;185:394-400.

[295] Enrique, E; Cisteró-Bahíma, A. Specific immunotherapy for food allergy: basic principles and clinical aspects. *Curr. Opin. Allergy Clin. Immunol.* 2006;6:466-469.

[296] Leung, DY; Sampson, HA; Yunginger, JW; et al. Effect of anti-IgE therapy in patients with peanut allergy. *N. Engl. J. Med.* 2003;348:986-993.

[297] Li, XM; Zhang, TF; Huang, CK; et al. Food Allergy Herbal Formula-1 (FAHF-1) blocks peanut-induced anaphylaxis in a murine model. *J. Allergy Clin. Immunol.* 2001;108:639-646.

[298] Li, XM; Srivastava, K; Grishin, A; et al. Persistent protective effect of heat-killed *Escherichia coli* producing "engineered," recombinant peanut proteins in a murine model of peanut allergy. *J. Allergy Clin. Immunol.* 2003;112:159-167.

[299] Mankad, VS; Burks, AW. Omalizumab: other indications and unanswered questions. *Clin. Rev. Allergy Immunol.* 2005;29:17-30.

[300] Okubo, K; Ogino, S; Nagakura, T; et al. Omalizumab is effective and safe in the treatment of Japanese cedar pollen-induced seasonal allergic rhinitis. *Allergol. Int.* 2006;55:379-386.

[301] Crespo, JF; James, JM; Rodriguez J. Diagnosis and therapy of food allergy. *Mol. Nutr. Food Res.* 2004;48:347-355.

[302] MacGlashan, DW; Bochner, BS; Adelman, DC; et al. Down-regulation of Fc (epsilon) RI expression on human basophils during vivo treatment of atopic patients with anti-IgE antibody. *J. Immunol.* 1997;158:1438-1445.

[303] Stein, ML; Collins, MH; Villanueva, JM; et al. Anti-IL-5 (mepolizumab) therapy for eosinophilic esophagitis. *J. Allergy Clin. Immunol.* 2006;118:1312-1319.

[304] Enrique, E; Pineda, F; Malek, T; et al. Sublingual immunotherapy for hazelnut food allergy: a randomized double-blind placebo-controlled

study with a standardized hazelnut extract. *J. Allergy Clin. Immunol.* 2005;116:1073-1079.

[305] King, N; Helm, R; Stanley, JS; et al. Allergenic characteristics of a modified peanut allergen. *Mol. Nutr. Food Res.* 2005;49:963-971.

[306] Peng, HJ; Su, SN; Chang, ZN; et al. Induction of specific Th1 responses and suppression of IgE antibody formation by vaccination with plasmid DNA encoding Der f 11. *Vaccine.* 2002;20:1761-1768.

[307] Horn, AA; Raz, E. Immunostimulatory sequence oligodeoxynucleotide-based vaccination and immunomodulation: two unique but complementary strategies for the treatment of allergic diseases. *J. Allergy Clin. Immunol.* 2002;110:706-712.

[308] Marshall, JD; Abtahi, S; Eiden, JJ; et al. Immunostimulatory sequence DNA linked to the Amb a 1 allergen promotes T(H)1 cytokine expression while downregulating T(H)2 cytokine expression in PBMCs from human patients with ragweed allergy. *J. Allergy Clin. Immunol.* 2001;108:191-197.

[309] Hsieh, KY; Hus, CI; Lim JY; et al. Oral administration of an edible-mushroom-derived protein inhibits the development of food-allergic reactions in mice. *Clin. Exp. Allergy.* 2003;33:1595-1602.

[310] Li, XM; Srivastava, K; Huleatt, JW; et al. Engineered recombinant peanut proteins and heat-killed *Listeria monocytogenes* coadministration protects against peanut-induced anaphylaxis in a murine model. *J. Immunol.* 2003;170:3289-3295.

[311] Srivastava, KD; Kattan, JD; Zou, ZM; et al. The Chinese herbal medicine formula FAHF-2 completely blocks anaphylactic reactions in a murine model of peanut allergy. *J. Allergy Clin. Immunol.* 2005;115:171-178.

[312] James, JM; Burks, AW; Robertson, PK; et al. Safe administration of the measles vaccine to children allergic to eggs. *N. Engl. J. Med.* 1995;332:1262-1266.

[313] Lacksman, R; Finn, A. MMR vaccine and allergy. *Arch. Dis. Child.* 2000;82:93-95.

[314] American Academy of Pediatrics. Allergic reactions to egg-related antigens. In: Pickering, LK; Baker, CJ; Kimberlin, DW; et al. (eds). *Red Book: 2009 Report of the Committee on Infectious Diseases.* Elk Grove Village, IL: American Academy of Pediatrics, 2009, pp.48-49.

INDEX

I

J

L

M